SOCIAL PALLIATION

Canadian Muslims' Storied Lives on Living and Dying

Social Palliation is a pioneering study on living and dying as articulated by first-generation Iranian and Ismaili-Muslim communities in Canada. Using ethnographic narratives, Parin Dossa makes a case for a paradigm shift from palliative care to social palliation.

Experiences of displacement and resettlement reveal that life and death must be understood as an integrated unit if we are to appreciate what it is like to be awakened to our human existence. In the wake of structural exclusion and systemic suffering, social palliation brings to light displaced persons' endeavours to restore the integrity of life and death. Dossa highlights the point that death conjoined with life is embedded within the socio-cultural and spiritual experience. Here, a caring society is not perceived in fragments, as is the case with traditional institutional care or care offered during end-of-life. Rather, Dossa draws attention to an organic form of caring, illustrated through the trajectories of storied lives. In exemplifying more humane aspects of social palliation, this book foregrounds sacred traditions to illustrate their potential to evoke deep-level conversations across socio-political boundaries on what it is like to live and die in the contemporary world.

PARIN DOSSA is a professor of Anthropology at Simon Fraser University.

PARIN DOSSA

Social Palliation

Canadian Muslims' Storied Lives on Living and Dying

UNIVERSITY OF TORONTO PRESS
Toronto Buffalo London

© University of Toronto Press 2020
Toronto Buffalo London
utorontopress.com

ISBN 978-1-4875-0523-3 (cloth)   ISBN 978-1-4875-3180-5 (PDF)
ISBN 978-1-4875-2530-9 (paper)   ISBN 978-1-4875-3181-2 (EPUB)

Library and Archives Canada Cataloguing in Publication

Title: Social palliation : Canadian Muslims' storied lives on living and
    dying / Parin Dossa.
Names: Dossa, Parin Aziz, 1945– author.
Description: Includes bibliographical references and index.
Identifiers: Canadiana (print) 20200305743 | Canadiana (ebook)
    20200305964 | ISBN 9781487505233 (hardcover) | ISBN 9781487525309
    (softcover) | ISBN 9781487531805 (PDF) | ISBN 9781487531812 (EPUB)
Subjects: LCSH: Terminal care – Social aspects – Canada. | LCSH: Palliative
    treatment – Social aspects – Canada. | LCSH: Death – Social aspects –
    Canada. | LCSH: Older Muslims – Care – Canada. | LCSH: Older
    immigrants – Care – Canada. | LCSH: Older Muslims – Canada – Social
    life and customs. | LCSH: Older immigrants – Canada – Social life and
    customs.
Classification: LCC HQ1073.5.C2 D67 2020 | DDC 306.9088297/0971–dc23

This book has been published with the help of a grant from the Federation
for the Humanities and Social Sciences, through the Awards to Scholarly
Publications Program, using funds provided by the Social Sciences and
Humanities Research Council of Canada.

University of Toronto Press acknowledges the financial assistance to its
publishing program of the Canada Council for the Arts and the Ontario
Arts Council, an agency of the Government of Ontario.

Canada Council   Conseil des Arts
for the Arts   du Canada

ONTARIO ARTS COUNCIL
CONSEIL DES ARTS DE L'ONTARIO
an Ontario government agency
un organisme du gouvernement de l'Ontario

Funded by the   Financé par le
Government   gouvernement
of Canada   du Canada

Canadä

بسم الله الرحمن الرحيم

Bismi Llahi Al Rahmani Al Raheem
In the Name of Allah, the Compassionate, the Merciful

Contents

Acknowledgments

This book would not have come to fruition without the generosity of participants who valued my research, were generous with their time, and graciously welcomed me and my research assistants into their homes and their lives. Their words and insights animate this book and my life. I am grateful to Lorraine Gerard, director of the BC Hospice Palliative Care Association, who introduced me to this project. Her support and encouragement have been invaluable. I benefited greatly from presenting and participating in annual conferences that she organized. I acknowledge the research assistants who collaborated with me, notably Rozina Janmohamed, Yasmin Popat, and Gulzar Shivji (the Ismaili-Muslim community); and Asa Rahmani, Poran Poragbal, Saba Azadi, and Golnaz Yazdi (the Iranian community). Casey Gray and Sarah Hein, recipients of the Vice President Undergraduate Research Award, worked closely with me as we collated data and conducted literature reviews. Simran Ahmed reviewed references for which I am grateful. I express my gratitude to Dr Muhammed Wardeh for the dedication and moral support. Thank you Ellen Hawman for your assistance with indexing.

For constructive critique of my work, I owe a debt of thanks to my colleagues and graduate students, notably Jelena Golubovic and Jenny Shaw. I also benefited from the comments received from presentations at conferences and workshops. My sincere and deep gratitude to the three anonymous readers from the University of Toronto Press. My deepest thanks to Jodi Lewchuk for her encouragement, guidance, and support. Special thanks to Barbara Porter and Gillian Scobie for their kind assistance and valuable input. I express my gratitude to Barbara for overseeing the publication process and to Gillian for her impressive and meticulous copy-editing of the manuscript. This research would not have been possible without generous funding from SFU's

Community Engagement Initiative grant, "From Knowledge to Collaborative Engagement: Inclusive Palliative Care for Immigrant Muslims"; a small SSHRC grant, "Coming of Age: Exploring the Needs of Elderly Racialized Minorities in Hospice Palliative Care in Urban Canada"; and the University Publications Fund.

My special thanks and gratitude go to calligraphic artist Khaled Al-Saa'i. His work represented on the cover and in the calligraphic illustrations of Rumi's verses speaks to his accomplishments. An award-winning contemporary Arabic calligrapher and painter, he has this to say: "One can select the style of calligraphy to fit with both the musical rhythm and the meaning of the selected poem or text, uniting them together as a whole. This is the key to generating new forms of art and the base from which we can create communication with anything."

My deepest and heart-felt gratitude goes to my soul mate and life companion, Aziz. Thank you for your continual support, encouragement, and trust in my work. Your love and unwavering faith have sustained me over decades of my ethnographic research, locally and abroad. As always, I have benefited from my conversations with my daughter Fahreen, a physician practising integrated health internationally and locally with First Nations. Software architect Louis-Michel Raynauld has been most helpful in addressing technological issues. Thank you for your time and patience. My son Zahwil and daughter-in-law Monika have been a source of inspiration, as have my grandchildren: Andre, Zoe, and Isaan. They have provided me with a much-needed break from my work. My life would not have been the same without the support and love of my family, including Yasmin Thobani and Khatoon Esmail. I owe a life-long debt of gratitude to my beloved mother, Nabat Khanu.

I respectfully acknowledge that SFU is on unceded Coast Salish Territory, the traditional territories of the Musqueam, Squamish, Tsleil-Waututh, and Kwikwetlem First Nations.

In Memoriam

دلی بی غم کجا جویم که در عالم نمی‌بینم

WHERE SHALL I FIND A HEART WITHOUT
SORROW, FOR I SEE NONE IN THE WORLD.
— SAADI, 1210–1291

IN REMEMBRANCE OF ALL THOSE WHO LOST THEIR
LIVES ON FLIGHT 752 IN IRAN, 8 JANUARY 2020

SOCIAL PALLIATION

Canadian Muslims' Storied Lives on Living and Dying

Introduction

I remember when I was in secondary school my mother took care of my grand-mother in Uganda. She was eighty-eight years old. She was sick and bedrid-den. We all knew that she was not going to live long. My mother said, "Allah will take her, when it is her time to die. It is not in our hands." Her bed was placed in the living room right close to the main entrance. Whoever came to the house whether they were visitors or the children back from school, we would all greet her. How could we miss her? She was right there. We felt her presence. Although she was sick and frail, she was a strong woman. She would talk to us and tell us stories even when she was not well. My mother said: "Seeing people and talking to them lessened her pain." She died peacefully as if she had chosen the time of her death. This was when we had come back from school and we were all present in the room. On the day she died, she had refused to take her medication. She knew that it was her last day and she wanted to be "awake." As an afterword, Jamila noted: "My grandmother taught us about life, dying and death."

(Jamila, 11 October 2016)

Contrary to our expectation that palliative care is a new phenomenon originating in the West, its deinstitutionalized existence in other cultural traditions requires acknowledgment. In today's world of advanced medical technology, what Jamila describes may be considered rudimen-tary. But this is a misconception. Without romanticizing home-based care, I would like to highlight some of the elements that we may want to revisit: the social visibility of the care recipient as opposed to them being confined to a room, fostering social relationships through kith and kin, and managing pain to the extent possible through self-care. In the case of the latter, I learned that Jamila's grandmother stretched parts of her body as a form of "exercise" to ease her pain. Home-based informal care may not be ideal. It has shortcomings, such as gender-based care and lack of "privacy."[1] At the same time, the grandmother's personhood was not diminished. Her physical and social visibility, her ability to share stories, and her control over the moment of her death are elements worth noting. The patient-centred focus of palliative care is premised on fulfilling the wishes of the patient as an individual, not as a person embedded in a world of social relationships (Dossa 2017, 193–4), and also as someone with a history and life experiences that should matter. The above anecdote helped me to think through my project as it evolved in conversations with interlocutors.

An ethnographer must have a good rationale for choosing a topic that requires intense and long-term interactions with study participants. I therefore asked myself what drew me to explore social palliation rather than palliative care.[2] My initial response was to foreground the paradox embedded in the latter, where patient-centred and compassionate care is contingent upon a diagnosis of terminal illness. I found this to be delimiting and unjust. None of the forty palliative care practitioners that I conversed with referred to this paradox. But my study participants, Canadian-Iranians and Canadian-Ismaili Muslims, occupying a socially marginal position as "first-generation immigrants," identified it in their own terms. Their responses took the form of broadening the parameters of palliative care through narrations of displacement and reflections on living and dying.

The relationship between living and dying was critical for the study participants. For them, displacement resulting from forced migration[3] had existential implications in the vein of what Zimmerman (2012) refers to as learning about ourselves through "the life and death of others" (220; also refer to Aries 2013). There is more to death than meets the eye. Death is not a discrete event. Neither is it an exclusively biological phenomenon. It is embedded in the socio-cultural, spiritual, and historical lives of people within which it is conjoined with life. The emergence of biomedicine (and its compassionate arm of palliative care) has, as Das and Han (2016) have argued, severed death from life; see also Garcia (2010), Gunaratnam (2013), Han (2012, 2016), and Ong (1995). *Social Palliation* engages with two interrelated questions: What bearing does displacement have on living and dying in a new land? And what kind of work do displaced persons engage with to restore the integrity of life and death, even if this is in small but not insignificant ways? I show that social palliation is closely linked with the conjoined unit of living and dying. The absence of one or the other undermines palliation. That is, social palliation does not fall under categories such as "best practices of care" or "culturally inclusive" palliative care.[4] Palliation assumed special significance for my interlocutors because their migration to a new place has led to the close relationship between life and death being severed, articulated through storied lives as well as the rhythms, sounds, and sentiments of sacred traditions with their potential to initiate deep-level conversations with stakeholders.

Scholarship suggests that the emergence of the biopolitical state, along with globalization and the neoliberal restructuring of markets, have cumulatively played a role in dismantling life from death. Displacement associated with ongoing ruptures constitutes part of this reconfiguration. It is in this context that Das and Han (2016) pose two critical questions that resonate with my work: "What is it for a human being to be awakened to his or her existence?" (2); and "How might we attend to the fragility of life, in the sense of a human form of life?" (3). The authors argue that we should become attuned to seeing how larger events "are nestled with the so-called small events and that it is their mutual braiding with each other that defines the texture of living" (6). Key questions that arose in my study are: how can we acquire a politically informed and palpable understanding of the stories that emanate from the marginalized space of displacement? In what way can we address the paradox by which affliction is perpetuated and medicalized by institutions established to relieve suffering in the first place? How can we read the words and storied lives of research participants to recognize them as producers of experience-based knowledge? What role do stories play in creating "a world we ought to know," to use Razack's (1998) term. These questions guided my analysis of stories along with sacred traditions speaking to the subject matter of life and death, with their potential to invoke deep-level conversations across boundaries.

Displacement is a politicized phenomenon that profoundly affects people's lives because they are compelled to leave their place of birth, after living there for generations. One would think that such a loss would be mitigated on arrival in the host country. This is not the case. Displaced persons are subject to continuing trauma. Displacement is largely a function of colonization and neo-imperialism (Abdelhady 2008; Abrego 2014; Bannerjee 2000; Brah 1996; Coe 2016; Colson 2003; Datta 2016; Long 2013). Therefore, we need to "attend closely to the complex and uneven reverberations and articulations in the presence of much larger historical geographies of colonialism and imperialism, along with their racialized as well as gender, sexualized, and ethnic forms" (Hart 2008, 694). Without overlooking the reality of internal displacement, it is important to note that, by and large, the flow of migration is from the global South to the global North and not the other way around. Upon crossing the border into the global North (the West), persons from the non-Western world are subject to a second form of "trauma" that interlocutors identified as non-recognition of their credentials and erasure of their life experiences, a function of structural exclusion.

Scholarly work on displacement puts greater emphasis on the political economy framework that uproots people in the first place and then provides minimal or no relief in the country of settlement (De Alvis 2004; Erel 2009; 2011, Gedalof 2007; Gilmartin and Migge 2015; Redclift 2016). Less attention is given to the political and social agency of displaced persons as they go about rebuilding their lives under challenging circumstances. A key aspect of this restorative work involves addressing the existential matter of life and death. As Fassin (2010) has expressed it: learning to live means learning to die. And death, as Stevenson (2014)) has argued, may be considered "as a passage of a new life" (131). Here, the human experience of living and dying (understood dynamically) presupposes the existence of another life; it also presupposes the existence of a home embodying this experience. Benjamin (1968) bemoans the way in which death has vacated our homes. "There used to be no house, hardly a room in which someone had not died. Today, people live in rooms that have never been touched by death" (94 cf. Stevenson 2014, 161). As I show below, when participants' ties with other people within and outside their dwellings were weak, they were rendered more vulnerable to their sense of being-in-the-world, where life and death are experienced simultaneously. Ethnography can come to our rescue as it reminds us to look closely at what human beings make of their lives and, equally, how studying their lives allows us to constantly question what it is to be human.[5] As noted above, the interlocutors of this study remained fully aware that life had to be lived in loss but not without remedial measures.

A central argument of this book, then, is to show that the severance of life from death has implications that cannot be overlooked. These implications make their way into the everyday lives of older people in particular, giving rise to sentiments of loneliness that my interlocutors experienced existentially. They feared that at the moment of their death, they might be alone – a fear that was shared by Allison's (2016) aging interlocutors. The issue is not that their families do not love them or care for them but that their families do not have the time to spend with them, and there is no way of telling in advance when the precise moment of death would occur. In a palliative care setting, family members took time off work to be with their loved ones, reasoning that their employers considered legitimate. Yet my observations revealed a deep contradiction embedded in palliative care. In this setting, dying with dignity can amount to inducing deep sleep through medication (hydromorphone), so that the dying person and family members can barely interact with one another. In the medicated state, when a person dies, he/she dies "alone," despite being surrounded by family. It is this deep fear of dying alone that the participants struggled with, and it is in this context that they sought to interweave life and death, connecting these two spheres in a world that considers them to be separate (Das and Han 2016).

Any work on life and death evokes human sentiments of frailty and finitude, but also of hopefulness. As Garcia (2010) has noted, we need to explore the question of how we can come to recognize that the suffering of others is our own. The aspect of shared pain and commensurability forms the subject matter of anthropologists such as Behar (1996, 2013), Crapanzano (2003), Das (2015), Fassin (2007), and Scheper-Hughes (1992, 1994). Each of these works focuses on how our seemingly separate vulnerabilities can be recognized and shared, provided we work through the structural barriers that separate "us" from "them." It is in this context that Fassin observes that we should think of "our shared humanity less in terms of difference than inequality; less as a matter of culture than history" (xv).

How people rework and reimagine their worlds is critical for this study. It is this dynamic between the political economy of de-/re-settlement and its localized reconfiguration that drew me to conduct ethnographic research within communities with whom I am familiar, and with whom I have long-standing ties, both professional and personal (Dossa 1985, 2004, 2009, 2017). The two communities I chose to work with are Canadian-Iranians and Canadian Ismaili-Muslims of South Asian origins. Long-term familiarity was not the only factor. These communities present an illustrative comparison, featuring both contrasts and similarities. Canadian-Iranians emphasize networks of social relationships, however diffused, between there (Iran) and here (Canada). For Canadian Ismaili-Muslims, *Jamat Khana* (the Ismaili word for mosque, literally translated as the house of congregation) constitutes the centre of their lives, so much so that families strive to live near one of the fourteen Jamat Khanas in British Columbia. The similarities rest on the two communities' common experiences of displacement. I am a South Asian Canadian Ismaili-Muslim. Hence, my familiarity with this community's language, socialization, and experience of displacement is more intimate than with that of Canadian-Iranians (Muslims and non-Muslims), with whom I have kept in touch since my earlier research in 2004 and 2009. For this project, I conducted sustained research with both communities from May 2015 to May 2018 in Vancouver, British Columbia.

Listening to the Voices of the Disenfranchised

Lambek (2016) has observed that societies have a tacit knowledge of dying and death. This was indeed the case with Canadian Ismaili-Muslims and Canadian-Iranian communities. Anchored in their sacred traditions, it was not unusual for interlocutors to cite verses from their respective traditions. Canadian-Iranians resorted to Jalaludin Rumi (1207–73), a household Sufi poet, among others, whereas Canadian Ismaili-Muslims cited verses from the Indian tradition of *ginans*, composed by *pirs* (wise men) in the eleventh and twelfth centuries. Recited every day in the Jamat Khana and informally by individuals, the *ginans* contain verses such as, "On the day of my death, call me and keep me close to you [the Divine Being] and hold my hand"; and "Live in a good way, you are definitely going to die." Verses from Rumi that I was privy to included: "You were born with wings, why do you prefer to crawl through life?"; "Don't grieve anything you lose. It comes around in another form"; and "There is turbulence beneath the surface." The appeal of these selected verses lies in their healing and aesthetic qualities; individuals cited verses to fill in empty hours or in the event of a crisis like illness or impending death. Being melodious and therefore more appealing, they were also recited to transmit to the next generation and tacitly for transformative change towards social palliation that addressed the interconnection between life and death. Everyday conversations were not bereft of the subject matter of life, dying, and death. But older persons noted that in the busyness of life, the younger generation did not reflect on this existential subject.

It is one thing to learn that death and dying are an integral part of one's life, and another to broach the subject in research. From the outset, I realized that it would be inappropriate to seek out families whose loved ones had been diagnosed as "palliative." Apart from the sensitivity of the issue, I thought that focusing on this sector would delimit my study in ways that would not do justice to the life experiences of people who had crossed geopolitical and cultural borders. As Gunaratnam (2013) has observed, "History, geo-politics, cultural and religious prescriptions hover around the migrant's deathbed" (8); this broader perspective transforms our understanding of living and dying, which I argue constitutes the foundation of social palliation. My previous work (2004, 2009, 2014) has alerted me to the importance of including alternative and non-conventional methods, such as memory work, the language of the body, the language of everyday life, and storytelling. The latter proved to be invaluable. As I have argued previously (2004),

> Stories must have a home in a community of listeners for whom the story makes a claim that will be remembered. The challenge here is to listen to the voices in a manner that allows us to capture the lived reality of the speakers while simultaneously to understand the shaping of this reality by the dominant system. Ultimately the task at hand is to recognize these women [participants] as producers of knowledge. (22)

The importance of stories is further noted by Pandian and Mariappan (2014),

> All of us come to life in a sea of stories. They sketch what we desire and fear. They take us back to times and places we thought were gone and to others that we've never imagined. Woven from many threads of our experience, they form patterns we didn't expect to see, directions we didn't expect to follow. (9)

Noting that we live in a fast-paced world, the authors continue, "Still, we need stories to make sense of this world and to judge how best to live with its challenges and possibilities" (10). Stories yield insights not captured in other methodologies. The literature on storied lives foregrounds the importance of staying with the stories rather than moving on (for example, Das 2007; Dossa 2004, 2014; Erel 2009, 2011). It is in this vein that Gunaratnam (2013) urges us to take time "to live with the stories and their affect"; they have vitality and musicality that bring them closer to ethics rather than mere methodology. An important aspect of the genre of storytelling is its close association with the wound (continual displacement). Emanating from the inner recesses of life, wounds tell stories that challenge us to reflect on aspects of lived realities that might otherwise recede into the background.

A compelling question that requires attention is, What happens to people who are subject to chronic illness and social suffering in contexts of structural exclusion and racism amidst a neoliberal state? The construct of social suffering lends itself to a nuanced analysis. To begin with, it captures the impact of structural forces on the lived realities of people. Second, one's suffering can be accentuated by the system that is supposed to mitigate its impact. Third, suffering can position people to exercise agency in ways that would not otherwise be possible. The experience of suffering enables people to foreground alternative ways of being, as was the case with study participants. Aging in the diaspora and being confronted with the issue of life and death, they sought to highlight the need for social palliation. This observation is of special relevance to my study participants, whose racialization within the nation state of Canada, imagined as white, rendered them socially vulnerable. Racialized minorities are not positioned to easily access the health care system, whose Eurocentric focus can be alienating and exclusionary (Agnew 1998; Anderson 1996; Anderson and Kirkham 1998; Spitzer 2011, 2004, 2015). Structural inclusiveness has not been systematically addressed by palliative care practitioners (Blevins and Papadatou 2006; Dilworth-Anderson et al. 2002; Fry et al. 2013; Williams et al. 2010). By and large, the practitioners with whom I conversed over the course of this research took the stance that structural inclusiveness was not an issue: "We do not distinguish between white, black, or anyone else. We take everyone who is referred to us as people and we treat them equally" (Karen); "If they have their cultural and religious practices, we accommodate them. The other day we had a drumming ceremony for a First Nations person. Twenty-five people came. We accommodated the ceremony, no problem" (Sophia). When I inquired whether other residents minded the drum beats or could benefit from the ceremony, the response was: "We have soundproof rooms. The noise does not go through to other rooms."

Drawing boundaries around socially categorized groups is debilitating from the point of view of learning about alternative ways of being and dying, not to mention the aspect of Othering by keeping "them" in "their" place and space. A walking tour that I undertook at three hospices revealed designated spaces for the performance of prayers and rituals. One hospice had a sacred room with icons that represented several religious traditions. Jennifer, the manager, put it this way: "A gathering of families and friends can be held in this room. All religions are accommodated." Two points require consideration: First, does the parameter *one size fits all* not gloss over the specific needs of communities, and the inequalities between them? And second, does the "blanket accommodation" approach not translate into drawing boundaries around cultures and traditions? The latter invariably Others people on the margins of society with the message, "You can do your own thing only within the space allocated to you" (author's summation).

When I stepped into the field, I realized that participants did not engage with the topic of palliative care. This may be because vulnerable people are less inclined to criticize the system. Furthermore, they considered the topic to be "too narrow" since it did not capture their life experiences or allow for an in-depth understanding of their struggles – the wounds they incurred in the process of living a life in a new land that did not welcome them except for their labour (Agnew 1197; Dossa 2004; Lee 1999; Li 2003); what was missing was society acknowledging their life course unfolding between nation-states and socio-cultural borders. More important, they felt that the prism of palliative care did not capture the integrity, however fragile and tenuous, of life and death. For the study participants, life could not be lived without an understanding of its intricate connection to death, and death would be devoid of meaning if it did not continue to inform the lives of the living. As Reimer-Kirkham (2012) observes, there are great disparities in access to meaningful palliative care:

> Current palliative care approaches do not make explicit the additional attention needed to address social and structural inequities that profoundly shape health, illness and dying experiences for people who are made particularly vulnerable by a constellation of sociopolitical, economic, cultural and historical forces. (215)

I argue that living, dying, and death, rather than biological facts subject to medical scrutiny, are phenomena that reveal what it is to be human in a world that is troubled and ripped apart by endemic violence and disruption of lives. I deploy stories and the sacred traditions (see Conclusion) with the goal of opening space for deep-level conversations across geopolitical boundaries. Here, it is vital that we create space for the intuitive knowledge and affect embodied in these traditions in a situation where "group typifications as a way of understanding the individual characterizes modern knowledge systems that operate through categories, codes and statistical possibilities" (Gunaratnam 2013, 104). Pain and suffering, as well as transformative change, cannot be articulated exclusively through language, a point of view advocated by Das 2015, Fassin 2007, Garcia 2010, and Gunaratnam 2013, among others. Das (2015) puts it this way, "Suffering that is assimilated within the normal and yet not fully absorbed in it is much more difficult to decipher … I want this term to lend itself to the environment and sensibilities that might sometimes call on God" (1). I believe that conversations, not only in the form of actively listening to what is said and what is not said, but intuitively grasped, constitute one means through which we can work towards social palliation – a caring society that acknowledges someone's life and border-crossing experiences. Study participants' experience of displacement translated into non-acknowledgement of their lives that, according to Cavell (1976), amounts to "active denial of the Other" (264). This situation is attributed to the workings of racialization (a process that study participants were subject to in Canada, their country of settlement), and exacerbated by neoliberal global capitalism, with its focus on autonomous individuals cut off from the existential concern of what it is to live and what it is to die.[6] A paradigm shift towards social palliation, I argue, would be enriched by being open to the rhythms, sounds, and words of sacred traditions.

The storied lives of my participants prompted the question, How was it that they felt isolated and lonely? Parents and grandparents did not consider their children to be solely responsible for this rupture. They internalized the discourse of the busyness of life and justified displaced care, claiming their children had tremendous responsibilities in raising their own families, providing for their well-being, and ensuring that they were attuned to their sacred traditions. One participant described this situation as treading on a fine rope. Parents and grandparents found themselves making all kinds of compromises and justifications, even concerning ritual ceremonies, such as reducing forty days of mourning to one week or even less. "Who has the time in this day and age?" This refrain surfaced in my conversations with participants. Yet there existed deeply felt anxiety that the participants sought to articulate. What would happen to them when they reached old age, when their health failed them, or when they were diagnosed as terminally ill? This anxiety was a new phenomenon for them. In their homeland, when a person was nearing death, through illness or old age, a support system, however inadequate, was in place even if this was an imagined scenario.

Widening the lens of palliative care, I wish to explore larger issues brought to light by the study participants, seeking to show that there is a whole person behind any kind of illness. By and large, my focus is on exploring continual displacement and its implications for how life and death are experienced. I would like to emphasize that displacement contains the seeds of transformation, mapped at the ground level by interlocutors – "geo-social politics from below" to use Gunaratnam's (2013) term.

Methodology

Having stimulated my interest in palliative care, the executive director of the British Columbia Hospice Palliative Care Association (BCHPCA),[7] Lorraine Gerard, suggested that I explore the issue of cultural and religious inclusivity. Lorraine provided me with the initial contacts that helped me to reach out to palliative care practitioners: physicians, nurses, frontline workers, and volunteers). I further learned who was who in the world of palliative care through platforms such as conferences, workshops, advertisements, and word of mouth. Over a three-year period, I conversed with forty practitioners, with formal meetings taking place in cafeterias, nursing homes, and hospice offices. I also engaged in limited participant observations at three hospices. I established contacts with members of the Canadian-Iranian and the Canadian Ismaili-Muslim communities through such measures as attending gatherings and festivals and community events, as well as by word of mouth. My previous work with the Canadian-Iranian community (2004; 2009) and the Canadian-Ismaili community (1985; 2009) helped me to refresh my contacts and establish new ones. Conversations with members of these communities took place at the following sites: homes, community or family gatherings (ESL – English as a Second Language, in the case of Canadian-Iranians), street walking, and cafeterias in Vancouver – my geographical field site. I continued my research over three weeks in May 2016 in Nairobi, Kenya, one of the home countries of the Canadian Ismaili-Muslims. Insights from this work enhanced my understanding of palliative care and the need to expand its boundaries.

The recruitment criteria were open. Families who wished to share stories of their lives were invited to participate. These stories invariably included concerns about health, ill health, and end-of-life in the context of what it means to cross geopolitical and cultural borders. One constituency that came forward from both communities was aging women, along with a few men. They came forward with the conviction that their life histories would speak to my research project on social palliation and not medical palliation; they felt that their wounds were deeper than what could be expressed in medical terms because, in the words of Shamim, "We have seen and lived more of life than our children." During my ongoing conversations with Shamim, she noted, "I am not referring to the length of time we have been in this world. I am referring to the life conditions that we have endured; our children will not know because they have not struggled like we have."

As a Muslim, my relationship with study participants from both communities was complex. For example, a terminally ill Canadian Ismaili-Muslim woman informed me that she would only talk to me if I did not approach her as a researcher. Hence, her story is not included in this work. I understood later that she wished to talk to me informally, as a "friend." Likewise, a Canadian-Iranian, also terminally ill, shared her life trajectory through her daughter, specifying that she wanted me to understand her situation so that I could offer prayers for her. Both participants relayed the complexity of research on death and the uncertainty of life, namely that discussion on such an issue does not fall under the rubric of insider-outsider; it calls for human interactions that participants emphasized as social palliation.

When they migrated in the 1970s, 1980s, and early 1990s, the participants were all in their forties and fifties. At the time of this research, they were nearing death in a new country where they were structurally excluded, as has been the case with other racialized minorities (Agnew 1996, 1997; Ahmed 1999; Bannerji 1993; 1995 Dossa 2004, 2009; Razack 1998; Thobani 2003, 2007). Structural exclusion delegitimizes one's life experiences and knowledge about life and death, but not to the extent of subjugating them altogether. Delegitimization can also strengthen one's resolve to rejuvenate what may be lost forever and go a step further. This context helps us to understand how participants' crossing of multiple borders (geographical, socio-cultural, and political) positioned them to engage in social palliation.[8] Here, living and dying is not understood as a discrete phenomenon but an existential issue tied to a way of life that participants had left behind.[9] Animated by participants' stories, I learned that in our grossly unequal world, social justice can best be addressed on an existential plane where life and death assume equal significance.[10] It was on this plane that participants sought to introduce social palliation.

I acknowledge the assistance of research assistants Rozina Janmohamed, Yasmin Popat, and Gulzar Shivji (the Ismaili-Muslim community); and Asa Rahmani, Poran Poragbal, Saba Azadi and Golnaz Yazdi (the Canadian-Iranian community). Casey Gray and Sarah Hein, recipients of the Vice President, Research Undergraduate Student Research Award, worked closely with me as we collected data and conducted literature reviews. Simran Ahmed reviewed references for which I am grateful. Each of the research assistants worked with me part of the time. To avoid the cumbersome task of referring to the nine research assistants, I have used the first-person pronoun throughout this work. The research assistants and I kept field diaries and made notes on informal and formal conversations that occurred in the course of my interactions with study participants, both palliative care practitioners as well as participants from the two communities. Out of respect, my visits to palliative care sites (homes, hospitals, nursing homes, and hospices) took place only through invitations from family members.

We conducted interviews in English with palliative care practitioners, Farsi and/or English with the Canadian-Iranians, and Gujarati and/or English with Canadian-Ismailis. Depending on participants' preferences, formal conversations were recorded and translated (where necessary). Alternatively, we (research assistants and I) resorted to note-taking if participants did not wish to be recorded. We paid attention to the nuances of body language, such as silence, and to the enactment of scenarios, such as tone, pitch of voice, and emphasis. I wish to state an unavoidable bias in the study. I do not speak Farsi and thus may have missed nuances that I was able to capture in Gujarati, my mother tongue. The names of all the participants, along with other identifying markers, have been changed in the interest of maintaining confidentiality (also refer to Appendix 1).

Social Wounding: Displacement and Re/De-Settlement

Social wounding reveals the dynamic interplay between estrangement and belonging, between being-in-the-world and falling out of it. The construct of social wounding helps me to underscore the point that the experience of isolation and loneliness, enmeshed in the everyday lives of older participants, must not be accepted as the norm. Social wounding suggests productive possibilities in the form of alternative pathways; wounds need to heal, given participants' concern that they would not be remembered in a way that would make a difference in the lives of their children and society at large. *Social Palliation* reveals an aspect of life that has been rendered ordinary when in fact it is *social wounding*. The issue at the core of social wounding is not that study participants are rendered passive. On the contrary, their attempts to re-make their everyday worlds are commendable. It is in this vein that they speak as *wounded storytellers* foregrounding singular narratives that perform a twofold task: revealing the effect of the structural forces at work along with their attempts at healing. The dynamic of singular and collective narratives captures the difference between wounded storytellers and social wounding, respectively. Their attempts take place in a world where individual-based activities replace the marked absence of meaningful social interactions. Mehrun put it this way,

> Our children tell us to keep busy. They bring us Indian movies to watch. They encourage us to read and go out. They tell us that this is the way to keep healthy and ward off dementia. We know all these things. We remain occupied. But we miss talking to people and getting a sense of comfort and security as we age.

The above observations prompt me to pay attention to the personal and the political, the intimate and the institutional. My goal is to show that everyday lived realities are intertwined with the politics of life that highlights "death-in-life" as a matter of course. As Garcia (2016) writes,

"Death in life is not a morbid manifestation that is somehow opposed to life but rather a vital experience that provides a basis for life's meaningful unfolding and even generates hope for the future" (316). My interlocutors were keenly aware of this observation as it spoke to their own lives, to posterity, and to society at large. In the context of palliative care, it means looking at larger scenarios beyond the confines of a clinic. Death-in-life evokes expansive questions on the meaning of life, relationally. Foregrounding the subjectivity of my interlocutors, I ask, How can we identify alternative modes of social life that reverse the condition of isolation and loneliness? In the context of this study, the pertinent question to consider is, To what extent does the condition of isolation contribute to life being severed from death? In other words, to fragmenting life? And how can this be remedied through social palliation? We may note the important work of Malkki (2015) – *The Need to Help: The Domestic Arts of International Humanitarianism.* Rather than being a one-sided relationship between aid recipients and humanitarian workers, Malkki illustrates the benefits accrued to the latter. She uses the example of elderly Finns to show how they mitigate their loneliness and need for societal recognition through their work of humanitarian handcrafts (knitting); the latter are a gift to themselves as it enables them to establish human connection and solidarity. Here, forming an imaginative community of knitters constitutes a therapeutic practice. We need to recognize the vulnerability of both the aid recipients and the aid givers. I argue that it is on this plane of the vulnerability of humankind, revealed poignantly in sacred traditions, that we can foster social palliation.

The importance of relationality of life-in-death and death-in-life was brought home to me during my visits to sixty-nine-year-old Shirin, who lives in an apartment complex in Burnaby, BC. As I stepped out of her sixth-floor apartment, I saw Kulsum, an older woman in her mid-eighties, walking up and down the corridor. I engaged her in conversation:

> I must maintain my health. No one has the time to care for me if I fall sick. This is the reason I walk. You know, back in Kampala [Uganda], I used to walk on my rooftop (*aghasi*). My daughter or my granddaughter would join me. I did not have to ask. The moment I went to the aghasi, they would come. I suppose they did not want me to be alone. We would talk, and it was our time to interact and exercise.

Kulsum's recollection describes a life in which exercising for health was not a discrete endeavour; it took place in the context of social relationships. Her solitary walks up and down the corridor speak to the fragmentation of her life, to the isolation these aging persons experience. This script, embodied in the image of an old woman walking by herself in the corridor, is connected to the structuring of society that results in what Allison (2013) refers to as "a lonely death," an outcome of a "relationless society" (663). I learned later from Shirin that Kulsum, who lived alone, was no longer taking her walks as she did not have the strength to do so.

Allison's work on elderly people in Japan offers insights that resonate with my work, and with what I understand to be my task as an anthropologist. She explores circumstances whereby "lonely dying/living produces a kind of suffering that in Elizabeth Povinelli's (2011) words, is ordinary, chronic, and cruddy rather than catastrophic, crisis laden, and sublime" (664). She asks, "What are the conditions under which people lose track of their elderly and are left, or leave others, to live and die unaccompanied by anyone else?" (664). Given scenarios like Kulsum's, which are not unusual, it is important to consider what Allison terms the "ecology of social belonging and care – and its apparent antithesis, abandonment and solitude – in life as well as in death" (664).

The integrity of life and death has been compromised in today's world where the politics of biomedicine is separated from the world of social relationships. Substantiating this point, Das and Han (2016) argue that the emergence of the biopolitical state has led to life being defined exclusively by biological knowledge, undermining social and spiritual definitions of human life. These need to be restored if we are to appreciate death as conjoined to life, rather than separate from it. Death can then be understood as part of social life (623). "Dying [then] is not something that happens to individuals but calls forth a response from all those affected by this process" (ibid.). "Response from all" and the way our lives overlap with those of others are attributes of social palliation.

The politics of exclusion that has taken the form of enclaving racialized minorities contributes to their isolation and alienation, and is barely noticed by the larger society. Racialized newcomers are expected to hit the ground running, as if their homeland lives and experiences do not matter. Commenting on how displacement can undermine one's being-in-the-world, Al-Mohammad (2016) puts it this way:

In the laboring of everyday life to secure a form of existence for oneself and one's families and friends, our lives overlap with the lives of others. The countless situations in which as persons and anthropologists we are faced with life projects that are struggling, however, suggests a greater dynamism to being-in-the-world since it is never an "account" that is settled, so to speak. Being-in-the-world does not mean one cannot fall out of the world we never held so securely. The world, though given to us in experience as the *given*, is nevertheless a *given* that can be taken, or simply fall away. (472–3)

It is the possibility of falling out of the world that brings home the reality of ongoing displacement, along with death severed from life. Repeatedly, I heard participants bring up the subject of dying, evoked by the death of a relative or a friend. The question they posed was framed in relation to the meaning of life, relayed through various scripts. If a well-to-do person passed away, the script revolved around the subject of wealth and how, ultimately, we leave everything behind. In the case of a young person dying from a terminal illness or accident, the script circulated among peers concerned the insufficient attention given to the fragility and finitude of life. The context of these conversations was the fear of becoming too materialistic and losing the intimacy of family life along the way, evoked by a participant citing Rumi, "I learned that every mortal will taste death. But only some will taste life."

In observing how study participants were struggling to make sense of their lives in a new country – struggles that resulted in participants reconfiguring their lives – I sought to explore how the larger forces, noted above, unfold in the everyday lives of individuals and families. As the participants aged or retired from the workforce, they came to realize that the lives they had endeavoured to build were fractured, a realization palpably expressed in loneliness and isolation, which cannot be overemphasized. Their immediate explanation was the busyness of their children's lives. Time and again, study participants told me that they felt they should not be a "burden" to their children, who already had too many demands on their lives. This constituted a reversal of traditional norms in Iran and East Africa (the homeland of the Ismailis) where parents could expect reciprocal care from children. One participant expressed this metaphorically: "We held their hands when they were young; now they can hold our hands as we age." I also heard positive stories of how children went out of their way to take care of and support their aging parents. Even in these stories, participants made comments such as, "but we do not know how long our children will support us. We pray that Allah gives them *shabudhi*" (ability to understand what is moral).

Aging parents expressed anxiety not only in relation to accessing care, but also in the context of everyday life; in the absence of social relationships, they felt that their lives remained unfulfilled. But this experience was not exclusive in the presence of subjectivity. As Biehl et al. (2007) expressed it, the latter "provides the ground for subjects to think through their circumstances and to feel through their contradictions, and in doing so, to inwardly explore experiences that would be otherwise outwardly unbearable" (14). In the case of study participants, subjectivity was evident in the multiple ways in which they remained occupied, such as attending exercise classes, watching preferred television programs, communicating with extended family members in the diaspora, shopping, cooking, and attending Jamat Khana (Ismailis) and / or cultural events (Iranians) to whatever extent possible. But these pursuits could neither fill the gap nor remedy the hurt they experienced in the absence of everyday sociality, translated into displaced care (Dossa 2018). Families and kin are what human beings count on for mutual support, care, and affection, notwithstanding expected conflicts. The rupturing of these networks took the form of a social wound. Although this wound profoundly affects the lives of those who experience it, it is rendered socially invisible. This is because the hurt and the suffering that originate from the wound are normalized in today's world. Yet social wounds do not remain passive. They speak and tell stories, as Arthur Frank (1995) has documented in *The Wounded Storyteller*.

Frank's use of the term "wounded storytellers," although confined to the experience of illness, connotes a layered analysis. First, he notes that wounded storytellers seek to recover their voices by shifting "the dominant cultural conception of illness away from passivity – the ill person as victim of disease and recipient of care – towards activity." He continues, "the disease that sets the body apart from others becomes, in the story, the common bond of suffering that joins bodies in their shared vulnerability" (xi). Second, he argues that the act of telling and listening is not easy, as "ill people are wounded not just in body but in voice. They need to become storytellers to recover the voices that illness and its treatment often takes away" (xii). Finally, wounded storytellers are ethically motivated to bear witness and become healers.

The wish to be remembered is a human condition. As Myerhoff (1980) revealed in her work with older members of the Jewish community in California, the need to be remembered was expressed in the form of rituals and murals that members hoped would be their legacy. They too felt forgotten as their children had moved away, and they were left to fend for themselves at a time when their health was failing them. The imperative to remember arises from a state of being wounded, whereby one bears the scars of social and political disorder that, in the case of the study participants, was the outcome of the violence of colonization, its offshoot of neoliberalism, displacement, and systemic racism, as discussed in the pages of this book (Razack 2012, 2008; Schepeur-Hughes 1994). Taking the stance of wounded storytellers, interlocutors positioned themselves to tell multiple stories in their own terms. This focus prompted me to listen deeply. This meant paying attention to how participants felt about the loss of interconnectivity in the wake of displacement, and how they made sense of their lived realities. The act of remembrance takes multiple forms that require researchers to pay attention to the small spaces within which memories are enmeshed: for example, among other things, a half-finished note, unfinished embroidery, or a recipe written on a scrap of paper.

Overview

This book will have fulfilled its purpose if it brings home the point that issues of life and death must be politicized. It will have attained its goal if it makes readers see that people have lives outside the space of palliative care that escape us because they are masked by depoliticized discourses of "compassion" and "dignity of life." Death is part of life, not severed from it. It embodies a complex web of relations, which encompass the politics of suffering and pain. Participants noted that when a person is no longer able to engage in meaningful social relationships and mutual interconnectivity, she/he is deprived of life at the fundamental level of experiencing its relationship to death. What enables us to see these connections are the life stories of people occupying different social milieux. People who are at the frontier of life and its evocation of death are well positioned to talk about life lived in space and time. This orientation contributes to highlighting our humanness, as to who we are, living lives that are finite and fragile. It is only in the world of social relationships that one can talk about one's experiences of life connected with death. One without the other does not capture the essence and the paradox embedded in living: the vulnerability and finitude of life and the certainty of death. For the participants, social palliation could not occur unless it addressed the question of what it is like to live and what it is like to die. They felt that their experiences of continual displacement positioned them to make a small contribution, effecting a shift that matters to us all: a conjoined unit of life and death embedded in a world of social relationships.

The chapters, I hope, capture what I heard, felt, and saw while being in the field and beyond; as my participants expressed it, "stories along with lived realities of life and death do not come to an end."

Chapter 1 lays out the parameters of the research context, as follows: (a) profiles of the two communities under study; (b) the culture and philosophy of palliative care in Canada; (c) a critique of "Privileging those who are already privileged"; (d) Islam and social palliation. Chapter 2 documents storied lives that participants relayed with the hope that this genre would capture their experiences of displacement that remain unknown and unacknowledged. Border-crossing moments along with everyday life are presented as key to understanding what is at stake as they go through the course of life, age, and prepare for death as part of life. Their insights on what it is like to be displaced and its bearing on life and death lay the groundwork for the rest of the book. Chapter 3 examines the dynamics of being-in-the-world and falling out of it. I draw heavily on the narratives of four participants whom I came to know well and who offered insights on precarity as a resource for living and dying. Holding on to the possibility of life folded into death requires close attention to the analytic of everyday life. I illustrate how forms of loss incurred through displacement are reconfigured, suggesting pathways for transformative change. This chapter introduces possibilities and contradictions in thinking about social palliation in relation to death-in-life and life-in-death. Re-making a home in the diaspora is the subject matter of chapters 4 and 5. As an anchor ground for life and death, I show how home is reconstituted precariously but also in relation to imagining alternative possibilities. My goal is twofold. First, I complicate the meaning of home, arguing that it is not a discrete unit unconnected to the larger world of border-crossings. Second, I seek to capture the humanity, vulnerability, and hopefulness of lives that I was privileged to know in contexts that are otherwise "dismissed" as mundane, not significant for societal change. In the concluding chapter, I explore the parameters of a shift from palliative care to social palliation. The pathway towards social palliation is what my participants desired. Speaking as wounded storytellers, they relayed their concern of loneliness and isolation that they felt could be remedied through sociality and inter-connectivity (social palliation) where their lives would be acknowledged. I argue that it is only when one's life is acknowledged that one can share the foundation story of humankind: what is it like to live and what is it like to die. I have thus organized this chapter as follows. In the first part, I present a summation of two narratives: (a) study participants, and (b) palliative care practitioners. In the second part, I briefly discuss neoliberalism, the context that has created a gulf between participants' understanding of life and death and the practitioners' focus on death as an exclusive phenomenon. To this end, I present fragments of the sacred traditions from the two communities (Canadian Ismaili-Muslims and Canadian-Iranians) in the third part. It is my hope that the repertoire of this rich heritage of life and death will create space for deep-level conversations with other traditions, thereby affecting a shift towards social palliation. My goal is to create space for reflection on the question raised by anthropologists, What are the forces that compromise our humanity taking into account differences that are valued.

PART 1

1 Research Context

"We are the Children of the Revolution": The Iranian Community[1]

What follows is a summation of the Iranian Revolution as described to me by my research participants. They attribute the cause of the 1979 Revolution to the over-Westernization of the country under the regime of Reza Shah Pahlavi (1923–78), as well as to the long-term "colonization" of Iran. This colonization did not take place through occupation, but by Russia and Britain appropriating the country's wealth. It is important to note that in 1953 the CIA instigated a military coup that ousted the popularly elected prime minister, Mohammed Mossadegh (Karim and Young 2006). Economic colonization does not occur in a vacuum. Along with it came a lifestyle foreign to the local people. People wanted change, but instead a theocratic and dictatorial Islamic government was ushered in under the banner of the revolution. This government is not what the people had desired (Higgins and Fischer 1981).

Scholarship suggests that the 1978–79 Revolution was sparked by a need for social justice. Vahabzadeh (2017) puts it this way:

> Iran's struggle for Social Justice has found its present shape through a collective sense of wonder: the Iranian Revolution, a revolution that at its core was a nationwide, popular movement for social justice and democratic self-determination, not a Shi'i state or Shi'i values, has produced, 37 years later, a sad reality contrary to the ideals of 1979. (1)

People who had worked for the Shah or were allied with him were persecuted. Young men were forcefully drafted into the army. Various social groups objected to the Islamization of the education system. The 1978–79 Revolution resulted in waves of migration as members of the middle class left the country to settle in the West, primarily in the

United States, Canada, and Europe (Farr 1999; Fischer 2010; Shahidian and Fathi 1992).

It was only after the repeated use of the phrase "children of the Revolution" by my participants in various contexts (conversations, social gatherings, and chatting on the streets) that I began to realize its importance. The participants conveyed the message that the goals of the Iranian Revolution – to restore democracy and freedom – had not materialized. In Canada, they hoped to restore the identities they had lost through Iran's over-Westernization, and to work towards establishing homes where they could maintain Iranian culture and traditions in relation to, and not divorced from, desirable Canadian values and practices. As Afari put it, the expectation was as follows,

> We have come here to establish a better life for ourselves and our children; we do not want to lose our traditions and our way of life totally [meaning that there would be some compromises]. Our lives were disrupted by the Revolution.

Encapsulating the sentiments of other participants, Afari continued,

> We have been on the North Shore for many years. There are minimal English language programs for us. They [the system] must have known that we are not all fluent in the language. We come from a country where language (*zabaan*) is part of our culture (*farhang-e Iran*). However "Westernized" we became, we did not lose our language. Now that we are here [in Canada], we need to learn English. I find that the European people are not accepting us. This may be because we [the Iranians] have chosen to live here on the North Shore. This area reminds us of the mountains in our country – the country that we left behind.

Afari concluded the above statement in a sad tone, on the verge of crying. She and her compatriots realized quickly that Canada was not the welcoming and accepting country that they had expected. Behi, Farnaz, and Golak, the women I met at the ESL classes, reported that when they first came to Canada, specifically to the North Shore, they felt very uncomfortable. "We did not stop on the street and talk to our friends [Iranian] as we felt that we would be judged" (Behi).

> You know the Iranians as they formed a community on the North Shore, they set up stores. The white people did not like this. They thought that we were taking over their neighbourhood. We were happy to have Iranian stores as it made us feel at home.

Some people are nice. When we go to the stores, they treat us nicely. But sometimes they also tell us off. Once I did not know that there was a line up for the cashier. Someone shouted, "This is not Iran."

Writing on Iranians who settled in the United States, Mobasher (2016) observes, "It can be argued that no other recent refugee or exile group has experienced the same intense, sudden sense of double loss or double exile and trauma that Iranians have" (26). This double exile and trauma refer first to forced migration, since families were compelled to leave their homeland to escape persecution, and second, to their reception when they arrived in Canada, which has been racist in every possible way: popular culture, settlement policies, the media, health and social sectors, and the labour force. To confront racist exclusion, Iranian women took it upon themselves to interrogate the systems of oppression and exclusionary practices, as I demonstrated in *Politics and Poetics of Migration* (Dossa 2004).

"Turmoil in our country brought us here." These words, which Mohammed uttered during a family gathering to which I was invited, were echoed by the study participants on various occasions. While each participant presented a singular trajectory of displacement, migration, and re-/de-settlement, within these individual narratives, the script of larger forces was invariably present. Some of the participants began their stories with the event of the Iranian Revolution, stating that it was brought about by the intervention of Western powers. Ali put it this way: "I wish Iran did not have the oil, then the West and Russia would not have plundered our country." Other Iranians referred to the way in which the Revolution had failed them, because the promised democracy remains elusive. Women were particularly critical of how the Revolution controlled them and their bodies, recalling incidents of being policed for improperly wearing the niqab. Some of the mothers I talked to observed that it was impossible to live in a country where their sons could be forcefully drafted into the army. Other respondents referred to the deteriorating economic situation, not to mention political oppression. They all highlighted the script of forceful displacement. Nazi put it this way, "If you ask Iranians and if they are honest, they will tell you that they would rather be in their own country (*mamlekat*) than here in Canada. The Revolution made it difficult for us to continue living there."

Iranians were aware that the process of displacement and dislocation does not end upon immigration but continues in the destination country. It results in further wounding at a deeper and intergenerational level, where it is rendered socially invisible. I recorded the following conversation between an aging woman (Marie) and a young volunteer (Parvaneh).

> MARIE: Do you know why I attend these classes? It is for socializing (*dor-eham boodan*). I learn some English, but this is not why I come here.
> PARVANEH: It is good that you are coming here. It gets you out of the house (*khane*).
> MARIE: I came to Canada twenty years ago. I was young at the time. I wanted to work. They [the system] did nothing for me. I was so angry. I told the immigration officer, "Why do you admit us into this country when you cannot give us jobs?" I am so isolated that I want to go back to Iran. But I cannot do that without my children.
> PARVANEH: I have been volunteering for the last five years. We have noticed that older people are isolated and lonely. I hope we can do something about this situation.

At this point, Sedigh interjected,

> Our children have busy lives. They do not have time for us. They phone me every day. When I ask them a question, they give short answers. The call only lasts for a few minutes. They really do not have time.

These observations bring to light familial issues and intimate matters, but embedded structural factors also need to be considered. Isolation and loneliness (*tanhaee*) are ultimately the result of the ethos of neoliberal global capitalism that requires younger people to adopt values of self-sufficiency and individualism – values that serve the marketplace, not the family. Wiegratz (2010) has argued that neoliberalism is not merely economic reform; it is a broader system of restructuring that involves "the cultural conditioning of individuals according to imperatives of capitalistic accumulation" (125). Referring to neoliberalism as an ethics of harm, Powell (2008) has made the powerful argument that "neoliberalism works by colonizing the field of values – reducing all social values to the market value" (177). She notes that this regime of power does not stop at this level. It simultaneously undermines social projects "by denying them sustenance" (ibid.). This sustenance, I argue, entails nurturing sociality vital to the well-being of societies – sociality that calls for an appreciation of the interweaving of life and death.

Conversations with other participants revealed that the values of individualism translate into the busyness of lives. Using the image of a cup of tea, Lamb (2009) encapsulates this point literally and metaphorically in her work on elderly American-Bengali immigrants. Her interlocutor pointed to the age-old Bengali tradition where older people are served an early morning cup of tea. Lamb observes that in India, you only have one cup of tea, while in the United States, you can have as many cups of tea as you like. The difference is that in India, you are served. In the US, you make your tea yourself. The difference between the two is substantive.

We cannot overemphasize the point that displacement is accompanied by a series of losses and disruptions: the loss of a familiar environment, the disruption of social networks, and the loss of a way of life and livelihood. The point I wish to emphasize is that human beings have the capacity to adapt to new environments; it is societal factors that impede one's attempts to rebuild a life. The women in my study worked hard acquiring Canadian qualifications while taking care of their families. As they approached the end of their lives, what these women desired was an acknowledgment of their struggles; to achieve recognition, the women in my study sought to posit a broader definition of palliative care, one in which acknowledgement is granted not at the moment of death, but in the context of a life course. In the process, they revealed that death is not a discrete experience; it is woven into life where it assumes the form of palliation, the core theme of this book.

The Ugandan Exodus: The Defining Moment for Canadian Ismaili-Muslims

On 29 August 1971, Idi Amin, then president of Uganda, announced that all Asians had to leave the country within ninety days. At first, the targeted population felt that it was a joke. How could close to 50,000 people leave the country within such a brief period? What about their livelihood, their children's education, and their family and community lives built over three generations? Realizing that the president had no intention of reversing the exodus edict, they began to accept the reality of forced displacement. Having lived under British colonial rule (1890–1962), the majority opted to settle in a Western country, such as the United Kingdom, Canada, or the United States, where they were desired for their labour and their presumed capacity to integrate into the mainstream society (Fernando 1979).

To be forced to leave a country within a short span of ninety days is traumatic. Rashida captures the sentiments of others when she says,

When I left my home country in such a hurry, I do not even remember what I left behind in my closets. I left behind so many memories that are lost. I remember one or two things at a time, like the gift of a handcrafted vase that my son gave me for my thirty-eighth birthday. What were the other precious things I left behind? Things that would help me to recall my life there.

The Asian exodus was a defining moment as it was during this time that the Asian Question loomed large, Were the Asians Africans or Indians (*muhindi* in Swahili)?[2] What was not considered was that the Asians' middle status position – above Africans and below Europeans – was created by the British colonial administration. It was essentially a divide and rule policy, the effect of which was far-reaching and structural.[3] In her work *Cartographies of Diaspora*, Brah (1996), who grew up in Uganda, observes,

> Looks mattered because of the history of the racialization of "looks"; they mattered because discourses about the body were crucial to the constitution of racisms. And racialized power operated in and through bodies. Moreover, racialized power configured into hierarchies, not simply between the dominant and subordinate categories of people, but also among them; that is between the "Indian" and the "African" in this instance. (3)

It is important to note that the Asians are not a homogeneous entity. Hindus, Sikhs, Parsees, and Ismailis, among other Muslims, were some of the communities who had made their home in East Africa. The Asians occupied a minority status that translated into vulnerability. The point of reference for each of these communities is India, their ancestral homeland. The distinguishing characteristic of the Ismailis is that they do not have a state of their own. By way of context, allow me to cite a paragraph from the scholarly work of Daftary (1990). (Also, refer to Daftary et al. 2015; Daftary and Hirji 2008a.)

> The Ismailis are a community of Shi'a Muslims who have settled around the world. Throughout their history, the Ismailis have been guided by hereditary leaders, Imams, who trace their genealogy back to the Prophet Muhammed through his daughter Fatima and his son-in-law and cousin, Ali. At various times in their long complex history, the Ismailis founded states, cities and institutions, contributed to the tradition of scholarship in Islam and were the patrons of learning and the arts. But the story of the Ismailis is also that of a religious minority who survived threats to their existence. Currently, the Ismailis are a pluralistic community led by their present Imam Shah Karim al-Husayni, Aga Khan IV. (2005, back cover)

H.H. The Aga Khan IV has directed the community to make homes in their various countries of residence. Accordingly, many Ismailis had considered East Africa to be their home. As my interlocutors informed me, their interpretation of this guidance meant contributing to their home country through hard work, service, and ethical living, ultimately leading to their being considered a model minority.

Other than assisting the colonial British to "develop" the East African territory along the lines desired by this regime of power, the Asians had no political or social status within what came to be known as the nation-states of Uganda, Kenya, and Tanzania, the borders of which were arbitrarily defined. Occupying a middle-man/woman status, the Asians benefitted materially: as "economic developers" they were structurally positioned above the indigenous African population and below the British colonizers. The vulnerability of this position came into sharp relief in the post-independence period of the 1960s. The newly independent states asked the question, Do the Asians belong to our countries? The government of Uganda took the official stance that they were outsiders, hence the decree to evict them even though the Asians had lived there for three generations, having been brought from India by the British as indentured labourers in the late 1880s. Kenya and Tanzania followed suit, not through drastic enactments but by advancing other strategies, such as a policy of Africanization that excluded Asians from multiple market sectors. Without a sense of home or belonging, many Asians left East Africa and migrated to the West hoping to start a new life. Their high level of education, along with their exposure to a Western/colonial way of life, gave them hope that they would be able to settle well in the West and establish a new home. This was not always the case. The project suggested by Brah (1996) for creating "new political subjects and new collective politics" (245) has yet to be realized.

The Western Agenda in Accepting Immigrants/Displaced Persons

The response to the question of the Asian settlement in the West is complex. First, we need to consider the political economy of migration. Imigrants are desirable because of their labour, both manual and professional, subject to their ability to integrate into the fabric of mainstream society. These are the criteria that inform immigration policies in the Western world (Agnew 1996; Bannerji 1995; Dossa 2004, 2009; Li 2003; Thobani 2007). Canadian Ismaili-Muslims met the criteria very well. Hence, they have come to be known as the model minority. Overlooked here, as I have demonstrated in my previous work (2009), are persons with disabilities and older people. Since they are not seen to head for the workforce, they are rendered socially invisible: a redundant population. Their marginalization has its origins in immigration policy but continues in mainstream society.

To reiterate a point made earlier, displacement amounts to a series of losses, such as the loss of a familiar environment and a familiar rhythm of life along with the loss of everyday sociality. All these elements are crucial for maintaining one's sense of being-in-the-world. In the context of struggles brought about by structural exclusion and racism, study participants informed me that they did not know how the years went by until they reached the iconic age of sixty-five, designating one as elderly. Some of the study participants told me that they were "forced out" of the workforce based on the unstated message that they had grown old and hence ceased to be productive, according to the standard set by fast-paced global capitalism. Others felt that their struggles were intense, and hence they chose to leave the workforce. Women who carried the double load of waged work and unrecognized household labour were hit hard. By the time they reached the age of sixty-five, their children had left home to establish their own nuclear families. They informed me that their married children and grandchildren cared for them but did not have time for them. The children were caught up in their own fast-paced lives. Cognizant of the societal neoliberal norms of individualism and self-care, these aging women and men did not want to be a burden to their children. Several participants told me that they would rather go into a nursing home than impose on their children. Intergenerational reciprocity and mutual care did not form part of this script.

Palliative Care: A Patchwork Quilt

In Canada, hospice palliative care (HPC) has existed since the beginning of the 1970s. It has evolved due to several factors: an aging population, increased longevity, a rise in chronic illness, and a shift towards community-based care (for example, Jack et al. 2011). Despite its commitment to the philosophy of patient-centred and compassionate care, the HPC model is embedded in the biomedical system, the primary focus of which is the management of the body (Lock 1993; Spitzer 2004; Seymour et al. 2007; Williams et al. 2010). Furthermore, the retrenchment of the health system under neoliberal restructuring has placed financial and systemic constraints on HPC at a time when it is needed most (Frey et al. 2013; Grande 2009; Williams et al. 2010). Faced with austerity budgets, advocates and health professionals have sustained HPC by circumventing the system, leading to what Williams et al. (2010)

describe as "a patchwork quilt." A closer look at the quilt reveals mismatched strands, not to mention omitted strands that would reflect the multicultural composition of Canadian society. Some strands connect with the biomedical model in which an illness vocabulary affirms one's patienthood rather than personhood. Other strands seek pathways of care and compassion but only within the parameters of palliative care. Regardless, patient-oriented care continues to be problematic because this focus, however well intentioned, reaffirms the neoliberal model of making the person responsible for his or her own well-being. This individualistic orientation places an enormous burden on the family at a time when they are about to lose a loved one. Adding other strands in the quilt could permit us to focus on holistic care: spiritual, cultural, social, and psychological (for example, Sharma and Reimer-Kirkham [2015] and Willis [1999]). But these remain submerged under the rubric of individualism and self-care.

While HPC is promising from the point of view of de-medicalization, realizing it in practice requires human resources that are critically lacking. HPC relies heavily on volunteers who work limited hours and are regulated by strict policies that determine what they can and cannot do. A volunteer who I came to know well put it this way:

> You know, we cannot work in a hospice setting without taking a course. I thought the course would be more humanistic to prepare us for interacting with patients and families. But I found that a large part of the course was concerned with rules. For example, we were told that we could not do hospice work if a close family member had passed away in the timeperiod of one year. I thought grieving for a loved one would help us to relate empathetically with the patient. I did not understand why they are so controlling.

This form of critique was hardly discernible in palliative care. Having attended three conferences organized by BC Hospice and Palliative Care Association (BCHPCA), along with two workshops, I observed that local politics of care in Vancouver (and other places in Canada) was not foregrounded. Keynote addresses and panelists talked about practitioners' "good and compassionate work." When I asked if concerted attention was paid to racialized minorities, the responses were invariably "we accommodate them on a case-by-case basis." There was no systemic approach to include them structurally; neither was there space for critical reflection.

Spirituality has been put forward as a viable non-medicalized approach to palliative care. Byrne (2007), for example, observes that "spirituality is essentially all about the essence of a person, and the first task for a spiritual carer is to affirm the personhood and identity of a patient" (118). This can be accomplished through validating care recipients' expressive concerns through such means as active listening and touching that would "expand our concept of language so that we hear, read and speak with our bodies as confidently as we do with our words" (122). This orientation can also be accomplished by acknowledging recipients' intuitive uses of metaphors, symbols, and narratives relayed in no small measure in sacred traditions. Consider the following verses from the ginan (*Ughmiyah sohi din athmiyah*) and Rumi's poetry, respectively.

Day rises, and the night comes
Flowers bloom and fade
Buildings are constructed and collapse
Those who are born will die[4]

There is a life-force within your soul
Seek that life
There is a gem in the mountain of your body
Seek that mine
O Traveller, if you are in search of that
Don't look outside,
Look inside yourself
And seek that

The conjoined unit of life and death constitutes the plane of social palliation; it is on this plane that people recognize their vulnerability, not overlooking the reality of inequality and injustice that makes some people more vulnerable than others (for example Das 2015; Farmer 2003; Garcia 2010; Gunaratnam 2013). Biomedicine is one area where this inequality unfolds poignantly. In her research on Cambodian refugees, Ong (1995) observes, "Among the schemes of knowledge and power regulating individual and social bodies, modern medicine is the prime mover, defining and promoting concepts, categories and authoritarian pronouncements on hygiene, health, sexuality, life and death" (1244). Foregrounding the Foucauldian viewpoint, she notes how biomedicine defines "social, economic and juridical practices that socialize biopolitical subjects of the modern welfare state" (ibid.). Ong does not overlook the subtle ways in which subjugated subjects reverse the biomedical gaze in small measures. A substantial body of scholarship shows how people on the margins exercise agency and creativity to negotiate systems of oppression (Boehm 2008; Dossa 2004, 2009; Gilmartin and Migge 2015; Hill-Collins 2005; Hintzen 2004). While acknowledging this counter-narrative, it is important that we address structural and systemic issues so that people on the margins do not have to engage in ongoing struggles with the system. It is tiring to be continually on the opposite side.

Within the biomedical landscape, palliative care occupies an ambivalent status. On the one hand, it has sought to free itself from a diagnostic, medicalized model of care. On the other hand, it is biomedical practitioners who determine the eligibility criterion for palliative care, and this care is administered in no small measure through drugs that are considered to advance a dignified and peaceful death. In this schema, the ideals underpinning palliative care are not fully realized, as noted in the words of its practitioners:

> Um, palliative care is, it's a philosophy that um … aims to, you know … like reduce the suffering of the patients as well as of the families. Patients are with illness and approaching the end of life. Improving the quality of life. Making sure that their choices and their preferences and wishes are respected as well as their needs.
>
> So, it's a holistic type of care. So, it's everything. It's not only the physical needs, it's the psychological, it's the spiritual, um and it is everything. Looking at the person, the patient as a person, not as a patient. Not only the medical or the health service needs, but also as a person. Um, so it's trying to help people you know, make a smooth transition to death by creating a comfortable atmosphere.
>
> I would say that palliative – palliation – is basically the provision of supports for people who are at the end of their life, when they are at the point in their lives where active treatment is no longer seen as an option. So, it's the, sort of the medical, spiritual and social care of the whole person as they approach the end of their life.

While palliative care practitioners seek to enhance the quality of life and personhood of "patients," a question that needs to be asked is, to what extent can this vision be realized within a short span of three months? In Vancouver, a person is only entitled to palliative care when he or she receives a medical diagnosis of death within this time-frame.[5] I consider this to be an anomaly as, fundamentally, life and death cannot be severed. In this book, I seek to broaden the parameters of palliative care where its temporal (time span) and spatial (hospice and hospital care) limitations could be reconfigured, creating "a pathway for reimagining human life as the mutual absorption of the natural and the social and the fragility with which they come to be aligned" (Das and Han 2016, 4). This orientation takes the form of social palliation (caring society) as opposed to exclusive palliative care (clinical model). Relationality and interconnectivity are the defining characteristics of social palliation. Citing Cavarero (2000), Stevenson (2014) makes the point that "a unique individual is not the atomized individual of modern political doctrines. Instead the individual is unique 'not because she is free from any other; on the contrary, the relation with the other is necessary for her very self-designation as unique' (89). The individual for Cavarero is constitutively in relation with others" (246). In her work on the lonely death in Japan, Allison (2013) observes, "the quality of being needed is the first and most common use of the word human" (8).

Privileging Those Who Are Already Privileged

Canada is one of the most culturally and religiously diverse countries in the world. Yet its health and palliative care system is premised on two founding (read: hegemonic) nations: the English and the French (Bannerji 2000; Razack 2012, 2014; Thobani 2014, 2015). The question, then, is, how do practitioners go about accommodating the diverse traditions of multicultural and multireligious communities without reifying them? It would not be an exaggeration to state that minimal work has been done in this area, let alone scholarship that addresses the complexities that inform our understanding of what constitutes culture, religion, and tradition embedded within diasporas rather than within the unit of the nation-state. Agnew (2005) writes,

> Diasporas thus denote a transnational sense of self and community and create an understanding of ethnicity and ethnic bonds that transcends the borders and boundaries of nation states. Yet, the individual living in the diaspora experiences a dynamic tension every day between living 'here' and remembering 'there,' between memories of places of origin and entanglements with places of residence, and between the metaphorical and the physical home. (4)

Commenting on the gendered strategy of empowerment adopted so that women can be equally included, Anderson (1996) makes the following points. First, she cautions us that well-meaning measures to promote the well-being of disenfranchised and racialized women can be deceptive as they do not take into consideration their lived realities. The women may not speak English, and even if they do, the discourse of the bureaucratic health system can be intimidating. Second, for disadvantaged women, the need for survival trumps managing illness. Therefore, Anderson writes,

> It would be misleading to conclude that knowledge alone determines illness management: even when a woman was knowledgeable, the material circumstances of her life profoundly influenced the management of her time schedules at work, exhaustion after work, family commitments – all impinge on her ability to manage an illness. (701; see also Dunn and Dyck 2000, Spitzer 2011)

A paradigm shift would occur, argues Anderson (1996), if there is

> Recognition of the historical factors that have shaped our institutions and the multiple forces of class, race, gender and other oppressions. *Until we unmask the unquestioned and taken-for-granted ideologies that are at the foundation of movements like self-care and that are interwoven into the seemingly liberatory ideas like empowerment [patient-centred care in palliative terminology], we will continue to produce "recipes for health and health care delivery" that privilege those who are already privileged and disenfranchise those who are dispossessed.* (703–4, emphasis added)

She emphasizes the point that,

> Achieving health is not just a matter of enabling people to take more responsibility for their health; it is also about managing injustice and taking action to address social and economic inequity. This will be the challenge of the 21st century. (Ibid.)

The terminally ill, I argue, are marginalized by the existing health and palliative care systems because of their exclusive focus on end-of-life. This phase of life, as I show in the following chapters, cannot be divorced from life, life that for the study participants entailed crossing geopolitical and social boundaries and re-making a home in a new land in the wake of displacement. This endeavour is rendered difficult not because human beings do not have the capacity to adapt to other socio-political environments, however different, but because of structural factors that impede adaptation. Here, history and socio-political locations come into play. How do these factors interface with palliative care? This question has not been addressed. Palliative care exists in its own orbit owing to its exclusive focus on end-of-life care. This explains interlocutors' reluctance to engage with this topic.

Ethnographers have long emphasized that major developments such as global capitalism do not descend unmediated into people's lives, especially those who are disenfranchised and displaced (Chatterjee 2009; Foley 2008; Misra et al. 2006; Yeates 2009). The latter's confrontation with the larger system that devalues them takes multiple forms that I do not dismiss as mere resistance. People exercise agency, but that does not mean that they are free from the pain and suffering brought about by a larger system that does not "see" them for who they are, namely people with histories embedded in moral and socio-political worlds. *Social Palliation* captures the dynamic interplay between agency and structural constraints through the conceptual construct of social wounding, manifested through the lens of continual displacement, along with its implications for life and death.

Islam and Social Palliation

The subject matter of Islam evokes two narrative scripts: Orientalism and its counter-narrative of diasporic subjectivities. The first one comprises the Western image of Islam as being irrational and uncivilized, and oppressive to women; this script was rejuvenated in the post-9/11 era when Muslims came under attack to advance the West's imperialist agendas, encapsulated in the invasion and military occupation of Afghanistan in 2001 and Iraq in 2003. Razack (2008) puts it this way: In the post-9/11 world, it is not just the so-called terrorists but also civilians, immigrants, and refugees who are categorically excluded from Western law and politics. She notes that race thinking justifies the treatment of Muslims as the Other; here, gender is used to illustrate the cultural flaws of Islam, the grounds on which the West assumes a superior status of being enlightened on women's rights while overlooking such abuses in their own countries. This presumptuous rationale motivated anthropologist Abu-Lughod (2016) to write *Do Muslim Women Need Saving?* (2016).[6] Rather than being a discrete entity, the subject matter of gender invokes entrenched inequalities based on race, religion, class, generation, and national heritage.

The second script, of diasporic subjectivities, is animated by the fact that Islam, a global faith with a diverse range of expressions and practices, is not contained within the politicized construct of the Muslims as the Other. Here, intersectional gendered contexts position women (not excluding men) to produce situated, imaginative, and alternative knowledges through interrelated arenas, such as everyday life (Liebelt and Werbner 2018; Selby et al. 2018); stories (Dossa 2014, 2019; Erel 2009, 2011); the body (Abu-Lughod 2016; Ahmed 2016); space (Dyck and

Dossa 2007; Rahder and McLean 2013); and, equally important, religiosity (Dilworth et al. 2007; Esmail 1998; Mahmood 2012; Reimer-Kirkham 2012; Sharma and Reimer-Kirkham 2015; Zine 2004, 2006, 2009).[7]

Faith-based/Islamic religiosity is of special relevance to *Social Palliation*. Three reasons may be cited. First, premised on the question of what makes us human, it forms part of the palliation landscape. Lest this question sound idealistic, consider what Ahmed (2016) and Fanon (1963), respectively, have to say. In *What Is Islam*, Ahmed calls upon the reader "to adopt a new language for the conceptualization of Islam" for a more nuanced understanding of the human experience at large (108). In *The Wretched of the Earth*, Fanon observes, "for Europe, for ourselves and for humanity," we must put forward new concepts that would result in the formation of a new citizen (316 cf. Isin 2012, 568). Anthropologists have long raised the question of what meaning human beings give to their lives, giving rise to further reflection on what makes us human. Second, in secularized countries, especially in the West, a faith-based perspective has come under scrutiny, so much so that it has been subjugated and invalidated; this is especially the case with Muslims, who have been subject to increasing surveillance and securitization in the wake of 9/11. By presenting a counter-narrative, Islamic scholars have highlighted religiosity as an avenue to reclaim their voice and representation of their lives and bodies. This body of discursive knowledge and practice has made it possible for women and men to narrate an alternative vision of what it is like to be a Muslim, not in a discrete sense, but in the context of the intersectionality of race, gender, religion, citizenship, and age. The paradigm of intersectionality creates multiple locations and strategies for mapping a possible way forward away from a clinical model of palliative care. It is important to note that the way in which Muslims foreground their understanding of Islam varies; contexts matter and so do particular moments and life trajectories. How they see the world and their place within it could form the groundwork for a politicized understanding of palliation. This third point requires a comment on the grounds that religiosity is not depoliticized; its embeddedness in everyday life (which includes discourses, spatial orientations, rituals, and sacred traditions) enables it to engage with issues of social justice and equality in ways that are subtle and nuanced. Translating these observations into the landscape of social palliation requires paying attention to the fact that religiosity is not always visible and easily accessible; it exists in the midst of powerful "secularized" ideologies.

Islam as a dynamic tradition and a religion, spanning temporally over 1,400 years and spatially across the globe, does not exist within its own orbit. It has invariably addressed societal concerns. Zine (2004) has aptly noted that knowledge of Islam "can enter academic dialogues and inquiries not as static dogma but as contextualized and historicized paradigm of thought that are referenced in metaphysical realities. They are not intended to operate as new grand narratives but, instead, can function in dialogical manner with other discourses and paradigms that may have a more secular foundation" (184). It is in this context that Islamic religiosity can shape the palliation landscape as an alternative vision that can ultimately enable us to reclaim our humanity based on social justice. This is the project that study participants sought to address from their respective locations, which included social palliation that they relayed through their storied lives.

2 Storied Lives

Storytellers strive to create a larger world of being and becoming, a world where they acquire a sense of belonging and where "their actions and words matter and make a difference" (Jackson 2006, 14). Stories enable us to assume the position of protagonists; they form a space that allows us to act as witnesses, to evoke a response from a listening audience. It is important to bear in mind that the most powerful and poignant stories emerge from the margins of society. Margins are spaces occupied by disenfranchised populations; their stories constitute the flesh and blood of life. They speak as wounded storytellers, to use Arthur Frank's term (1995). As I have noted earlier (2009), stories must find a home in a community of listeners on whom the stories make a claim to be remembered. Our challenge is to listen to the voices of the protagonists in a manner that allows us to capture their lived realities while simultaneously understanding how the dominant system shapes those realities. Most important, stories enable us to share "human predicaments of how bodies of all kinds survive frailty and loss and through interdependence" (Gunaratnam 2013, 22), a core theme informing social palliation.

The act of storytelling assumes the presence of other people, an audience through which one can "*imagine* that one's life belongs to a matrix greater than oneself, and that within this sphere of greater Being one's own actions and words matter and make a difference" (Jackson 2006, 14, emphasis in the original). The act of reaching out sustains a sense of agency in the wake of disempowering forces, reconstituting events so that they are reworked "both in dialogue with others and within one's own imagination" (ibid., 15). It is through this form of dialogue that we feel that we are "actively participating in a world that has otherwise discounted and demeaned our lives." And "[T]here is no denying that storytelling gives us a sense that though we do not exactly determine the course of our lives we at least have a hand in defining their meaning" (ibid., 16–17).

The imperative to engage in storytelling is greater when the world does not acknowledge our social existence and fails to recognize our worth as human beings. Stories are then "authored and authorized dialogically and collaboratively during sharing one's recollections with others" (Jackson 2006, 22–3). Hence "the story comes into being within an already existing web of human relations" (ibid.). Ultimately, then, the need for stories reflects our desire "to be part of some kindred community" and "this need is most deeply felt where the bonds of such belonging are violently sundered" (33–4). It is through storytelling that we can claim some sense of agency and purpose. It has the potential to "call into question our ordinarily taken for granted notions of identity and difference, and so push back and pluralize our horizons of knowledge" (25). In this sense, storytelling is like any other speech act in which the force of language derives not from its own internal essence or logic, but from the social and institutional context in which it is deployed and authorized. Through storytelling we strive to show that our personal world relates to the wider world of the others, "so that one's voice carries and one's actions have repercussions in the state, nation or community with which one identifies" (25). Our task then is to recognize the narrators as producers of context-specific knowledge. It is only at this level that we can speak with them and not for them, that is, to speak in the mode of conversation and not appropriation.

In this chapter, I ask: what kinds of stories emerge from the margins of society? As noted in the introduction, the margins that I draw from are inhabited by displaced people seeking to address the existential matter of living and dying. Their concern is that they will be dying in a country far away from their homeland – a country where they have not been able to settle down beyond the material level embedded in the market economy. Hence, their stories call forth an understanding of a full life course that, in the case of study participants, entailed the intertwined processes of colonization, displacement, and re-/de-settlement.[1] Death does not occur in isolation from lived life. At issue here is how life is lived, not at the time of crisis but in the context of everyday life. It is this point that study participants sought to convey. *Social Palliation* illustrates the multiple ways in which storied lives bring home the need for a caring society that understands the need for social palliation because of its concern for the lived experiences of social suffering. The latter requires us to pay attention to images and narratives with their capacity to evoke emotional responses while prompting critical reflections on social inquiry. It is in this context that Biehl (2005) focuses on singular narratives while tracing the harm produced by structural forces (also refer to Das 2015 and Gunaratnam 2013).

The above observations lay the groundwork for exploring the storied lives of three racialized women: a Canadian Ismaili-Muslim woman, Saker, and two Canadian-Iranian women, Nazi and Goli. I chose not to demarcate the two communities through separate chapters. Instead, I wish to highlight their commonality through the prism of displacement, re-settlement, and end-of-life as it unfolds throughout a lifetime, not just at the moment of death. Each woman's experience is markedly different from that of the others but, ultimately, they foreground a collective narrative on what it is like to live and prepare for death in a "foreign" land. Each of the women seek to affirm life beyond death so that they can be remembered within a web of social relationships. Saker was rendered a refugee in her homeland of Uganda, a place from which she was evicted, along with other Asians. She lived in a refugee camp in England where she later settled for seven years. After this, she was "displaced" a second time, immigrating to Canada and starting over yet again. Nazi's and Goli's experiences of displacement were brought about by the 1978–79 Iranian Revolution. Both women were compelled to migrate for family reasons – Nazi for her children's education, and Goli to be with her children. All three women struggled in a new place not because they were unable to adapt, but due to external barriers that determined their lived realities. A function of structural racism, such barriers, which Das (2015) refers to as the "corrosion of everyday life," cannot be easily named.

Each woman relayed her story with references to her homeland, a significant move because homeland experiences and memories are not acknowledged and given recognition in a country like Canada, where immigrants are expected to integrate and hit the ground running (Agnew 1996; Dossa 2009; Li 2003). Posing the question, who is a Canadian, Thobani (2012) observes, "Perceptions of 'Canadian-ness' and what it means to belong to the nation as a *Canadian* are deeply political and cultural. While those individuals and groups perceived as 'more' Canadian are imbued with greater cultural and political entitlement, those seen as 'less' Canadian are constantly constrained by and reminded of their 'immigrant' status regardless of birth or citizenship" (vii). Study participants used a counter-narrative as they sought to establish a connection between here (country of settlement) and there (homeland). Foregrounding a politicized script of displacement and re-making of home within ruptured spaces, they engaged with the question, what is it like to live and what is it like to die. The singularity of the stories does not diminish their collective significance: the stories

speak to the subject matter of ongoing displacement and its implications for social palliation. Ultimately, these are human issues, existential
moments we all share, that must not be looked upon as wholly other.

Saker: "You have thrown me here with the *dhodlyas*" (white people)

These are the words that Saker uttered within five minutes of being
admitted into a nursing facility. Without having yet interacted with the
staff or residents, Saker already sensed that the place she had come
to live would perpetuate the isolation she was subject to in Canada.
What were the circumstances that led her to stay in a nursing facility
for a period of four years, after which she passed away? She was not
ill. Other than mild dementia, Saker was healthy. How does a relatively
healthy person end up in a nursing home? Researchers have highlighted
multiple paths for placement. Some of these include being rendered a
widow or widower, not wanting to live with children owing to different
world views between generations, or to children's mobile lifestyle. At
issue is the embeddedness of these factors within the larger narratives
of globalization, modernity, and neoliberalism (Ayers and Saad Filho
2015; Foley 2008; Ganti 2014; Misra et al. 2006; Yeates 2005). Each of
these narratives is geared towards the market economy model with its
orientation towards individualism and self-care. Garcia (2010) observes
that in neoliberal regimes, the family bears the burden of care. I would
argue that this burden extends to the individual as well. This is the
larger context that accounts for Saker's placement in a nursing facility.

My meetings with Saker took place at four sites: her home, the cafete-
ria, Jamat Khana, and the nursing facility. In our first meeting, I asked
her if she wanted to share her life story. "We have come into this world
to share. Maybe my story will help others to pay more attention to the
lives of older people." It is on this note that she relayed the following
account.

Zindagi Chalti Hatih: Life Was Flowing (before Displacement)

Over *chai nasta* (tea and snacks), Saker observed that in her affinal
home in Kampala, Uganda, *zindagi chalti hatih* (life was flowing). She
explained that there she raised three children, cooked for an extended
family, stitched clothes for the women folk, socialized with visitors,
and, most important of all, visited Jamat Khana. This was the place that
gave her peace and absorbed the sorrows that she felt married women

often go through. "You know," she noted, "when you live in a large family, the pots make noise" (there is bound to be conflict). Compared with her life in Canada, Saker was happy in Uganda.

> It was my home. I knew my neighbours. I used to walk to Jamat Khana. I knew the streets. I would visit my children's schools to see how they were doing. There was always some occasion or festival that we celebrated. My life was hard as I worked the entire day, but it was good. I remember a house full of people. Here, in Canada, life is not bad, but I feel *lonely* and *alone*. Whom can I tell? My son is always busy with work and his family. I have two daughters: one lives here and the other lives in Calgary. Daughters are *parku dhan*, meaning their responsibilities are towards their in-laws.

Saker's selective reconstruction of her homeland life should not be perceived as nostalgic; her recall of a life lost through the violence of displacement is politicized. Sugiman (2004) reminds us that nostalgia has a liberating potential; it permits some escape from a coercive present by revisiting a better past. For the study participants, the past and the present were lived in two different countries and two different contexts: the global South and the global North. The latter subjugated and colonized the former. Participants emphasized the point that they would not willingly have left their country of birth, except that they were coerced to leave. Saker evokes the past not only to make sense of the present, but to highlight what she considers crucial for humankind, namely the world of social relationships. "I remember a house full of people." Saker makes this observation with the full knowledge that in her country of settlement, this everyday scenario from the past has become a rarity. She sees her task as that of creating a social world, as its presence in her current life is minimal. It is this very absence that makes her revisit a scene from her past.

Flipping through the album that she had packed in one of the two suitcases that Ugandan refugees could take with them, she paused at a picture in which she and her younger sister are seated on a swing:[2]

> This swing makes me recall my carefree days in my father's house in Masaka (a small town in Uganda). I was very happy, but my biggest regret is that I could not study after grade seven as there were no schools beyond this level.

When Saker was growing up, Uganda had long been colonized by the British (1894–1962). Saker's inability to continue her education was a function of the colonial bias towards "developing" urban centres, in this case Kampala, where infrastructure and services for rural areas were overlooked. As an alternative, Saker's father encouraged her to take up sewing, a skill in which she excelled.

> When I got married, life was not that easy. No one laughed in our house. It was just work. I cooked for eight people. In the afternoon, I stitched clothes for all the women in the house, including my mother-in-law. The best part of my life was when I went to Jamat Khana. I never missed a day as it was walking distance from our house. All three of my children would go with me. I went early so that I could do volunteer work. I set up the place, making sure that everything was in order for the ritual ceremonies and for worship. I encouraged my children to study as I knew that this was the best gift I could give them. Sometimes in the afternoons, I would go to the stores to pick up the fabric. On the way, I visited my friend for tea and talk. This was my time out. This was my life in Kampala, the city where I moved after marriage.

Saker's world was not ideal, but it was nevertheless a world in which life was flowing (*zindagi chalti hatih*). This world collapsed following the 1972 Ugandan Asian exodus. "We were given ninety days to leave a country that had been my home." How she must have felt is echoed by Moti Bai, a female protagonist in Somjee's (2016) work, *Home between Crossings*. Upon hearing of the impending exodus from Kenya, Moti Bai observes,

> That night in bed I clutch my *tasbih* [rosary], and at once begin rolling it. The fear of my slipping confidence in the President, then in the country and finally in myself overwhelms me. The fear of my children's tomorrow grips me. The shock and distress of exodus plagues me. No prayer words come to me, yet I keep moving my *tasbih* [rosary]. The feel of each bead passing through my fingertips calms me, for fingers on tasbih carry memories of peace. (296)

Moti Bai's observation is of interest. She is wounded from having to leave a country she has called home until middle-age. And yet she finds solace in a small but not insignificant act, "fingers on tasbih carry memories of peace." Saker recounted her departure as follows,

> We had taken up citizenship of Uganda. We wanted to live in this country. But we had no choice. When you don't have a choice, then the people who take you in [namely, the British Government] also do not give you a

choice. My two daughters left for Canada as there were rumors that girls would be forced to stay in the country to marry Africans. When we went for the interview, we informed the British embassy that we would like to join our daughters in Canada. They said *"No"* [emphasis in the original], you will be better off in England. They allowed my in-laws to go to Canada because a family friend had agreed to take care of them. My husband, my son and I were sent to a camp in the countryside. We lived in the camp for over three months. I kept myself busy. I organized the evening prayers for my community [Ismaili-Muslims]. I passed my time, helping other people, like bringing food from the kitchen for an older woman or getting milk for a pregnant woman. I heard other women saying, "She is like a horse. She walks so fast." I like to keep busy.[3]

As I got to know Saker, I began to realize that she was seeking out and working towards fostering social relationships. She was creating a world integral to which is social palliation whereby people notice who you are, reciprocally. When she went to Jamat Khana, Saker wore a big smile, greeting everyone, even people she did not know. Her life in her country of birth was embedded in relationships, even if not necessarily ideal and not always of her making. Nurturing social relationships has a bearing on the integrated unit of life and death. It is in this world of people that conversations take place on matters such as health, illness, care, and death. Such conversations bring home the reality of death by evoking discussions on moral issues, such as how one should live and the legacy one would want to leave for posterity. Woven here are the poetics and musicality that solidify human relationships through aesthetics, morality, and emotive content, which are expressed substantively in sacred traditions. These are significant so we can understand how the trajectory of life unfolds over the course of a lifetime, ending in death, as opposed to viewing the latter as a discrete reality to be managed medically. This theme is salient in Saker's life story.

The eviction of Ugandan Asians was inseparable from the colonial violence that rendered them vulnerable. Recruited by the British to develop the territory of East Africa, the Asians participated in the building of the East African Railway and opened up *dukas* (stores) in the interior. The British positioned the Asians as middlemen between themselves and the Africans, using the Asians to deter the Africans from attempting to climb the economic and social ladder, undermining, in multiple ways, the African identity and way of life. It was no coincidence that after the British left, the Africans vented their frustration and anger on the Asians, who had made a home in the East African countries of Uganda, Kenya, and Tanzania for three generations (Dossa 1985, 1999). When the British admitted Ugandan Asian refugees into *their* country, they positioned them to advance their economic agenda. That is the primary reason why immigrants and refugees from so-called developing countries are admitted into the West (Agnew 2005; Lee 1999; Li 2003). As Saker's narrative illustrates, no consideration is given to their personhood, who they are, and the world they have lost, and how they can go about rebuilding their lives.

"My Home Was in the Beautiful English Countryside"

Saker, her husband (Amin), and their son lived in the camp for three months, after which they were given a home in "the beautiful English countryside," as she put it. At first, she appreciated the spring flowers, the rolling hills, and the greenery – the scenic beauty reminded her of her homeland country of Uganda. It did not take her long to realize that she was in a golden cage (*sonanu panjaru*).

> Soon after we had a home, both Amin and I were offered jobs in factories. We worked from 8:30 in the morning until 5:00 in the evening. All that I had to do was pack candies. This is not difficult work, but to do this for a whole day was tiring. They [the store staff] were very strict and gave us very short breaks. There were barely any social interactions. After work, I went grocery shopping and filled two bags. At times, the bags were heavy, and I carried them in the bus. When I came home, I cooked and afterwards cleaned the kitchen. We said our prayers at home. There was a makeshift Jamat Khana but it was far. We could only go there once a week when my son could take time off from school. There were no other Asian families close by that we could connect with. That was my life for seven years. I felt we were in *sonanu panjaru* (a golden cage). We were materially comfortable but there was no social life. What kept me going was visits from relatives. Our siblings and their children visited us from time to time. They too were displaced Ugandans. They lived in different parts of Great Britain as well as in Canada. My house was always open for them. I prepared special meals when they came over.

Saker leaves it to the reader to imagine what it is like to be displaced. One of her compatriots, Malek, put it this way,

> We were made to work like donkeys. We did not even have time to look around as to where we were going with our lives (*zindagi*). Years went by

so quickly that I felt that I lost a good part of my life. Yes. We were earning. We could afford goods and make our lives comfortable. But there is more to life than *ash aram* (material comfort).

When I visited Farida, also a compatriot, I was struck by her contemporary furniture and her kitchen, fully equipped with all the modern gadgets. Responding to my comment on her beautiful home, she said, "I find this all very artificial." Both women lived in England and later migrated to Canada.

Having worked hard for close to three or four decades, most of the study participants were materially secure. Their children were doing well and were in lucrative professions. Even so, participants felt that their lives remained unfulfilled, and as they aged, they realized that they did not have long to live. The awareness of death constituted part of the very act of living, a flow of life imagined as "soul, life force, spirit, energy or animation" (Lambek 2016, 643). The participants' understanding of the flow of life was articulated as *jivan* (life) and *maranh* (death). The realization of the latter was expressed in the form of the refrain, "Do not forget to pack your *bhatu* (food) now for the long journey that will begin when you die." The packing of bhatu cannot take place in isolation. Its preparation requires virtuous deeds, generosity, and kindness – qualities that call for the active presence of other human beings. The dearth of this opportunity translates into living a life of isolation and loneliness. This was Saker's experience that she sought to convey through the story of her border-crossing life.

"For us, as we age, loneliness (*akulsadu*) is a major concern"

While Saker was in England, she sought to make a home away from home. She prepared breakfast and packed lunches for the family. She shopped and cooked in the evenings and made special meals when she had visitors. During weekends, she worked in the backyard of her two-bedroom house. In the spring, she planted roses and some vegetables. It was during this time that her English neighbour chatted with her.

> I felt so nice being able to chat with my neighbour. In some ways, it was strange, as I felt restrained at times. In Kampala talking to the neigbours (*padoshi*) was a done thing. It was part of everyday life. Here, it appeared to be strange talking to her only when I was in the garden. I never got to know her, but the conversations helped me with my English.

Saker did not know any English when she left Uganda. She acquired a functional knowledge of the language through her everyday interactions – largely utilitarian – at work and while shopping.

As time went by, Saker began to feel that she was missing out on what mattered most to her: attending Jamat Khana and having regular contact with people. When her son Rahim graduated as an engineer and got married to a nurse, she encouraged him to move to Canada. It was not a difficult move for the couple because of their qualifications. After two years, Rahim sponsored his parents, an application that went through quickly as family sponsorship requires the applicant to provide support for a period of ten years.[4] It is important to note that Canada's immigration category of family sponsorship classifies aging and older people as dependents; overlooked here is their kinship work including childcare, cooking, nurturing, and fostering cherished cultural values, along with numerous unrecognized everyday tasks (Dossa and Coe 2017).

When Saker and Amin migrated to Vancouver in the mid-1990s, they encountered a situation that they had not envisioned: the lifestyle of their own community had changed in keeping with the prevailing trend towards nuclear family units. Instead of living all together, Saker's son rented an apartment for his parents, ensuring that it was close to Jamat Khana. Saker lived in this dwelling for fifteen years. During this time, her son and her married daughter were her primary caregivers, since they were her only family in town. Her second daughter, who lived in Calgary, visited her regularly. As Saker aged, she began to feel lonely. Consider the following example.

It was a wintery day when Saker and I met at a coffee shop close to her house. She suggested that it would be a good place to chat. I did not realize it at the time, but she made her suggestion because it was a long weekend and she was feeling lonely. Her son had gone out of town, her daughter was busy with her in-laws, and her husband had passed away two years before. She noted that her children did not realize how lonely she was feeling. They visited her, brought her food, and picked up groceries for her, but they did not stay for long. "They have busy lives and I cannot expect them to spend too much time with me. I need to occupy myself." When I asked her about her everyday life, she observed,

> When I get up, the first thing I do is say my prayers. Then I have my breakfast. After that I read for a while and then have my bath. Twice or three times a week, I go to the mall by bus. Even if I do not have to buy much, I just walk around a bit and then go home. Riding on the bus is

nice as I see people, especially elderly people. I feel that my situation is the same as theirs. In the afternoon, I catch the news and watch T.V. Around 5:00 p.m., I get ready to go to Khane [short form]. The Jamat Khana bus picks me up.

As Saker went through the routine of her everyday life, I noticed the absence of people. Except for short visits from her children, she has barely any contact with other people. She may have a quick conversation with the cashier at the mall, but this is mostly utilitarian. Her significant connections take place in Jamat Khana where she meets friends and acquaintances, but even this is only for a brief period. This is because the bus departs soon after Jamat Khana is over.

"The hearth fire will not be extinguished"

Amin, Saker's husband, did not participate in our conversations. But on the topic of food (*khawanu*), he noted,

> When we were in England, I would come home late. When I saw my wife in the kitchen, I had a tremendous sense of *shanti* (peace) knowing that I was not coming into an empty home. This was nourishment for my body and soul. When we came to Canada, I felt the same way. Seeing my wife cooking made me feel that there was *someone* to take care of me.

Amin's emphatic tone on the word *someone* is telling; it suggests that the network of family members who would have been around to care for him as he aged had been diminished to only one person: his wife.

Saker had a different take on her role in the kitchen. She evoked a scene from back home when "women would cook together for a large family." It is interesting to compare this comment with her earlier account of life in Kampala, in which she relayed the point that she was the only one who was cooking for a large family. Presenting a different script in her country of settlement, Saker seeks to foreground a collective scenario of togetherness and sociality – a scenario that does not exist anymore. Echoing Saker, other participants also relayed memories of how cooking together fostered everyday interactions in their home country. In Canada, the women's discussion on cooking revolved around engaging in piecemeal tasks determined by their work schedules; for example, soaking lentils at night, boiling them before heading to work, and doing the *vaghar* (adding spices to make a curry) once they returned from work. Other women talked about mixing all the ingredients and resorting to using the microwave to save time.

Saker ensured that "the fire of the hearth was not extinguished," though it may have dimmed. She continued to cook for her family even when she lived by herself after the death of her husband. She explained that her children's lives were pressurized, and that cooking a dish or two would make life easier for them. One particular dish that she was skilled at making and that she continued to make for a long time was *rotis* (unleavened bread roasted on a special pan/*tawdih*). The importance of rotis can be gleaned from the fact that in East Africa they were a staple part of meals; some women brought tawdihs with them when they migrated to Canada. Consider the following vignette:

Making Rotis (Unleavened Bread)

It was 10 a.m. when I arrived at Saker's apartment. She opened the door with sticky hands because she was kneading flour for rotis. She had chosen this time for our visit in response to my question about her everyday routine, saying "Come to my place and see what I do." Realizing that she had too much dough for one person, she explained: "This is not just for me. My son will be visiting on Saturday and my daughter will be coming by on Sunday. I am making a lot of rotis so that I can share these with my children." Making rotis is time-consuming, and it is an art. Once the dough is kneaded, it is divided into individual portions. It is then patted with a bit of oil and a sprinkle of flour. The sides are folded, and each roti is rolled into a round shape. It is then cooked on the stove in *tawdih*. Saker was making twenty rotis.

> I will eat a few and the rest I will freeze. My children will visit me over the weekend. I will share the rotis with them. We do not always sit down and eat together. They do not have the time. They will bring me some food that I freeze, and they will pick up the rotis. They are always in a hurry. They have so many responsibilities. They are working and taking care of their young children.

A scene from back home portrays a different image. Saker's children informed me that in Kampala, their mother would often be in the kitchen when they came home for lunch. As the family sat down for dinner, she or their African maid would bring hot rotis to the table. Considered a staple food, eaten with a meal or as a snack, rotis were ubiquitous. What does it mean when in Canada rotis are made in the spirit of maintaining a traditional practice, yet are not eaten hot in the presence of family? Instead they are frozen to be eaten according to individualized schedules. What is the impact on the everyday life of an older person eating home-made rotis all alone? Saker's attempt to keep the tradition alive is commendable, and although it is ruptured, it must be recognized.

Rotis evoke memories of home. Participants recalled the past, how when they got back from school, their mothers would be making rotis on a charcoal stove, to be eaten hot with butter. The warmth of this dish reflected the warmth of a home where their mothers took care of them. Sixty-six-year old Farida had this to say,

> It was a comforting feeling. When we came home, we imbibed the aroma of rotis, fresh and warm. This is how our mothers took care of us. Those days are gone. These days, who remembers what parents and especially what mothers do for their children?

She made this comment in a group conversation on how the world has changed in the wake of individualism, integral to a lifestyle informed by neoliberal capitalism that is premised on self-responsibility and self-care.

Saker showed me the special roti pan that she had brought with her from Kampala. Although she does not use it anymore, the pan enables her to reconstruct her life when she prepared food for a large family, as opposed to making rotis for a family that is no longer intact. For Saker, the kitchen was a site of social activity.

> I did not just cook. When a neighbour would drop in, I would make tea. We would sit and chat. When children came home for lunch, the first place they came to was the kitchen where warm rotis awaited them.

Lest Saker's reconstruction of this memory image be considered nostalgic, I would like to reiterate that the recall of such images is politicized because they serve to identify discrepancies between the past, and the here and the now. A major gap that Saker and her compatriots identified was the feeling of loneliness and isolation; she makes rotis for the family, but they do not have the time to share them over a meal. The irony of this situation should not be lost. At work are socio-political factors connected with the market economy that leave little time for adult children to spend with their elderly parents.

Plaza (2014) writes,

> Our early food socialization leaves deep marks in the ways we perceive, relate, consume, and imagine a sense of "home" in the world. The power of food as communication resource, as site of narrative performance, and as mediator in cultural encounters is particularly important for immigrant communities. (469)

Imagining a sense of "home" in Canada is a ruptured experience for Saker and her cohort. Her children are around, but they are not fully available at critical times, such as mealtimes. It is within this ruptured space that Saker works to ensure that the fire of the hearth is not extinguished. It is also within this ruptured space that she thinks she will be remembered after death. "It is after one dies that children remember their parents," she observed several times during our meetings. It is interesting that she uses the impersonal term "one" and not "I." How is it that a person living in isolation and filling in empty hours can gain a sense of certainty that he/she will be remembered? I noted this point on the margins of my diary.

For Saker, the space of the Jamat Khana was an extension of her own kitchen and home. Initially when she cooked, she would keep aside a dish to take for *nandi* (prayer food). She impressed on her children that prayer food leads to abundance (*barakat*) and peace (*shanti*). The long-established tradition of taking nandi to Jamat Khana symbolically translates into sharing food with the community. It connects an Ismaili home to the Jamat Khana and by extension to the community. The food is placed on a low table (*pat*) and then taken by a family through the process of biding. The ties established with families that one does not always come to know serve to create a sense of solidarity. Later, as she aged and was unable to cook nandi, Saker would take store-bought food such as milk, fruit, or cookies. Improvisations of this kind ensured that the "fire of the hearth" – the source of familial solidarity – was not extinguished. Its flame remained even when Saker found herself, against her will, in a nursing home. Whenever I visited her, she would state, "You must have some tea. What can I give you to eat?" Although she could not serve food in the material sense, this gesture of sharing formed an important part of her tradition.

Life-in-Death

As Saker aged, she began to experience falls. Being a resourceful person, she would crawl to a chair and use it as a support to get up. At times, she used the telephone to call her Ismaili neighbour, the only person she knew in the apartment block where she lived. Most of Saker's falls did not hurt her much, but in one case she was hospitalized. It was during this time that a nurse brought up the subject of sending her to a nursing facility. Saker put it this way, "She told my children that they are very busy. They would not be able to take care of me in my old age. She told them that they should think about placing me into a home." Reflecting on the nurse's words, I thought that her advice was not well thought out. The health care system did not make provisions for the nurse to learn about Saker's life as an immigrant woman. Her life history would have revealed her resourcefulness in settling down in two different environments – an English countryside and a Canadian urban centre. The fact that she had lived on her own, taken care of her family, and done service work all her life speaks volumes about her ingenuity in making a life despite the constraints of language and the lack of a support system. Yet the nurse saw Saker as a woman who had frequent falls, not as a person who could take care of herself with some support. The nurse's recommendation was based on "the norm" that children are busy with work and with their own families. Taking care of older people is not seen as equally important. More significantly, the reciprocity of care, whereby Saker had continued to serve her family, did not come into play.

Saker's placement in the nursing facility was a tremendous shock for her. She said, "You have thrown me with the *dhodiyas* (white people)," meaning that she felt she had been placed in an alien world. This heartfelt statement speaks to the larger story of the ghettoization of racialized minorities. Except in the workplace, newcomers barely have the opportunity to interact with established residents. I observed that study participants invariably made a distinction between "Canadians" and "us." They would often say, "Canadians do it this way and we do it differently. Their children leave home at the age of eighteen. This is not our way." Saker found herself alone in a world that she had not envisaged in her wildest dreams: a nursing home whose residents were "white," except for one Ismaili-Muslim woman who passed away shortly following Saker was admitted. Saker had not had the opportunity to interact with that group before she was admitted to the facility.

During my numerous visits, she would tell me, "I am in a prison. This is the place where I will die." The busyness of her children's lives meant that her cries for help were not heard; neither were they heard by the health care system.

In the facility, Saker took to walking the corridors calling for her parents, her in-laws, and her brothers, all of whom had passed away. An otherwise alert woman, her mental health deteriorated in a situation where she was defined solely as a "demented resident." McLean and Leibing (2007), among others, take issue with such a label. They argue that although dementia has now been medicalized, it was a natural part of aging before the 1970s. In a nursing facility, this condition is exacerbated due to the excessive focus on disturbed behaviour, which is controlled through medication.

If we were to focus on the lived realities of people, we would realize that so-called disturbed behaviour has much to offer by way of fresh insights. Saker remembered her home in the small town where she was born. She remembered, "There was a swing, and me and my sister loved it, sitting together and pushing ourselves up and down, up and down." These were the carefree days of her life. After marriage, she felt that her in-laws mistreated her made her work hard. Yet she recalled pleasant moments, like picking jasmine from the garden to make garlands that she would take to Jamat Khana. The scent of jasmine remained with her, as she would often say, "You give a flower to someone, but the scent remains with you." Recalling her life, she reflected on how she would encourage all her children to study; in the case of her two daughters, she would not allow them into the kitchen, stating, "Go and read. This will help you with your education." She continued to update her telephone contact book containing the names of her relatives. My count showed over fifty names. Sadly, as she was reaching the end of her life, Saker was reduced to a resident with a room number. She would ask her children to take nandi to Jamat Khana on her behalf – fruit and milk, symbolically and socially nourishing. And whenever I visited her in the nursing home, she would insist that I have chai. A gesture of her enduring hospitality – the flame in the hearth.

Saker felt that her personhood was nullified when she was admitted to the nursing facility. Yet she presented a brave front, for example sending nandi to Jamat Khana or compiling a family tree through the phone numbers of extended and scattered members of the family. When she passed away, her family members stated, "She is in a good place"; "She is at peace"; "She was such a good woman; it cannot be otherwise"; "I feel her presence all the time." These words consoled them and perhaps helped them to accept their hasty decision to place her in a nursing home. If we were to ask Saker, she would have said these words masked the wounds she incurred at the nursing home. These wounds need to be recognized in relation to the story of her life: her courage, her resourcefulness, and her tenacity in re-making a home across multiple borders. Who she was and what she was reduced to must not be forgotten. The story that her wounds tell brings to light larger issues that I reflected upon after returning home from her funeral.

Having been privy to Saker's life, I remain convinced of the "moral imperative to speak up," otherwise we "fail to see how life slides into non-life," to borrow Das's words (2015, 169). The failure to reflect on what has been rendered socially invisible undermines our sense of what it is to be human. The question is, how do we go about addressing this issue? My response is to consider the foundation story of humankind:

the integrity of death-in-life and life-in-death. I argue that such an awareness fosters social palliation because it emphasizes existential issues: life and death. Saker's narrative reveals her brave attempts to sustain death-in-life, not only through the story she shared with me, but also through the way she lived it. In the process of living her story, she revealed how under difficult circumstances she had kept *jivan* (life) and *maranh* (death) in the forefront. She would often say, "We are going to die. We must live our lives with this awareness." Such observations, as Stevenson (2014) has argued, allow us "to formulate a robust image of how life, death and language are connected" (131). To implement this call, we need to be connected to a world of social relationships/palliation that Saker tried to revive within ruptured spaces.

Nazi: "I helped others to overcome their isolation. Now in my old age, I feel alone and isolated."

Nazi is one of the participants among several others whom I met first when she came to Canada in her late forties, and established contact with again when she was older. My first meeting with her took place at an ESL class (2002), a program that she helped to set up for aging Iranian women. She lives in a North Shore apartment complex populated by Iranian families. Like others in her cohort, she was subject to the deskilling process as an immigrant: although she is fluent in English, her credentials as a teacher were not recognized in Canada.[5] Once, as we were chatting after class, she informed me how satisfying it was for her that Iranian women attended the three-hour class twice a week. "They stay for extra two hours just to socialize." She proudly recalled how an encounter with an older Iranian neighbour convinced her to organize ESL classes. Her neighbour, Afari, used to go for walks everyday by herself. When she was no longer able to go for walks, she traversed up and down the corridor of her second-floor apartment. This was her way of "going out" to mitigate her loneliness, which had become a ubiquitous part of her life. Nazi felt that this was an experience she could relate to. As she explained,

> These women, regardless of whether they are widowed or not, must fend for themselves as their children are busy. They do not want to be a burden (*mozahem*) on them. But then loneliness (*tanhaee*) affects their well-being. They did not seem to be happy. I had to act.

Nazi approached the director of a senior centre and suggested that they set up an ESL program for Iranian women. While the director liked the idea, she informed her that the centre had no funding. Using an emphatic tone and gesturing with her hands, Nazi said,

> I did not take no for an answer. I embarrassed them by offering to work as a volunteer teacher. After eight months of service, the centre agreed to fund the program. They gave me a small salary. I did not mind. I set up the program to get older people out of their homes. I saw that they were becoming depressed, and *no one was asking about their health* (emphasis in the original). It was not just about learning English. It gave them the opportunity to socialize. You must have noticed how they stay on for one or two hours after the class is over. They need to have the opportunity to just talk.

The women used the space of socialization to celebrate birthdays and births as well as the festival of *Nurooz* (New Year). On these occasions, they brought cakes and Iranian sweets to share with everyone, including non-Iranian volunteers. During this time, conversations revolved around their homeland as well as their country of settlement, as they shared stories about familial and larger events. Haleh, a participant, expressed it this way,

> We learned so much from our interactions as to what was going on in both the countries. Talking about what was happening and what we remembered about this place made us feel that our ties with our homeland were not broken; and yet we realized that we had to build a life (*zendeghi*) here too, but not by leaving out our culture and the values we grew up with.

Officially, ESL classes are set up to integrate newcomers into Canadian society. The emphasis is on positioning them to join the labour force. As Bonny (2000), Bannerji (1995), Dossa (2004), Razack (2008), and Thobani (2007) have noted, racialized minorities do not enjoy substantive citizenship rights; they are accorded the status of the Other. Their way of life, culture, and traditions are not fully recognized. This point was captured by Shaheen, an ESL participant: "My teacher tells me that I should speak English at home. How can I do this? If I speak English at home, my grandchildren will grow up without knowing Farsi." Sara, who was part of this conversation, noted,

> Why don't they educate white people to talk to us in English outside this class? We go shopping, we have white neighbours, but these people hardly talk to us. We could learn English if they interacted with us. This way we can continue to use Farsi with our grandchildren. We want to learn English, but we do not want to give up our own language.

Lack of recognition of plural languages amounts to what McCarty et al. (2011) refer to as "the normalization of 'standard' English homogeneity" (35). They argue that this "is a key ideological mechanism in structuring social linguistic inequality" (ibid.). It is important to emphasize that language acquisition entails more than learning words, grammar, syntax, and pronunciation. Languages embody memories, worldviews, and traditions. The erasure of one's mother tongue at the cost of learning a new language leads to estrangement, for example between Sara and her grandchildren, if they grow up without speaking Farsi. It is desirable that newcomers become conversant with the languages of Canada without having to abandon their own language. Sara used this conversational moment to highlight a larger issue: the lack of opportunity for her cohort to interact socially outside the private space of the home. Nazi felt that ESL classes should serve as a springboard for further informal conversations between established residents and Iranians. Such opportunities, she noted, were few and far between.

Ironically, in her old age, Nazi finds herself facing the same situation that she sought to address for others: loneliness and isolation.[6] She unhesitatingly states, "I helped others to overcome their isolation. Now in my old age, I feel alone and isolated." She is a widow and lives by herself in an apartment complex on Lonsdale, a street in North Vancouver. Her two daughters are married and have moved to Toronto with their husbands. She informed me that when she is well, she goes for walks. Once, I accompanied her. Although she meets some Iranian people on the street, their interaction is limited to small talk, barely extending beyond polite greetings. The young people she meets are in a hurry, and those whom she befriended at the ESL classes are not around. Many of them have passed away, she tells me, and others have gone back to their country. She explained, "Their families send them to Iran if they cannot take care of them."

Nazi is a resourceful person. She tries to keep herself busy by reading, cooking when she can, and watching Iranian and Canadian television programs. But her health is failing her. She has arthritis, which she feels will become increasingly debilitating. She worries that a time may come when she will not be able to go out at all. She imagines a life filled with loneliness and empty hours. Although she manages to keep herself busy, she realizes that her family is not around her. She feels elated when, twice a year, her daughters visit with their children. Although one of her daughters has invited Nazi to move in with her, she declined because she does not want to be a burden. "They have busy lives, and they have their children to take care of as well." It is only when Nazi is in pain that she speaks from her "invisible wounds," relaying the message that she helped others to escape loneliness and depression, and yet now, in her old age, her experiences are no different from those whom she assisted.

I was impressed by Nazi's resilience and her ability to keep herself occupied. She would collate family photographs of her parents' siblings and their children living in different parts of the world, including family members who have passed away. Like Saker, she too is engaged in constructing a family tree. She thinks that this is important as her children do not know all their relatives and have not had the opportunity to meet family members whom they left behind, decades ago. She has begun to write her life story and has continued her passion for reading. One area that she focuses on is health and well-being – home remedies as well as allopathic ones. She identifies the most relevant information to share with her daughters "as they do not have the time." Nazi feels satisfied that she will leave a legacy though she cannot overcome the harsh reality that she is alone in her old age while struggling with arthritis. Having visited other aging Iranian women in a similar condition, I wondered if it is morally right to normalize a situation in which people are left to live alone while their experience of loneliness and isolation remains unnoticed by the larger world. These experiences form part of social wounding, which the participants sought to bring to light by relaying their stories. Such experiences constitute the crux of continual displacement, suggesting a pathway for change towards palliation.

Nazi lives in a social world where older people are rendered redundant, a situation that is compounded for aging racialized persons. The assumption at work is that their multiple contributions to Canada are minimal. In the logic of the market model, their tangible and intangible work remains unacknowledged: the work of assisting their families to settle down, along with their work in nurturing cultural traditions, however ruptured the process may be (Dossa and Coe 2017). Nazi is keenly aware of how people are displaced in Canada as well. During our conversations, she would often comment on the unfair treatment accorded to older persons from other countries. Once, as we were sitting in a café, an older Iranian woman, Kobra, walked in. She greeted us and sat at the table next to us. Nazi struck up a conversation with her and asked her if she was waiting for someone. She replied, "I am waiting for my son. He dropped me at the doctor's and asked me to wait here. It will be one or two hours before he can pick me up." Commenting on her situation, Nazi stated, "This is not uncommon. Children are so busy." Later, she noted,

> Did you see how well dressed Kobra was? Most of the older Iranian women dress up after breakfast. It gives them the feeling that they are going out. But they do not have the opportunity to go out. They might do some shopping. They are lonely day in day out. This is the reason why I set up the ESL program.

On one of my visits to her, she told me, "A human being should not have to experience loneliness (*tanhaee*)." As I was to learn, this aspect comes into sharper relief as one ages, a time when people seek social connectedness, when they seek to feel wanted and recognized as persons who have lived a life with all its trials and tribulations.

Nazi is worried that a time will come when she will not be able to go to out to shop, to do her banking, or to see her doctor. Her arthritis, she feels, is getting worse. Towards the latter part of our meetings, she began to talk about her husband, who "left this world just a few years after we came to Canada. He was not keeping well. May Allah rest his soul in peace." It was this information that made me realize how brave and courageous Nazi was. This is because in her homeland, Nazi would have had kith and kin that she could count on for support, not just nostalgically. As she explained, "they would just be around and help if they could." When I asked her if she had friends that she could turn to, she stated, "They are my age and they have their own issues. I cannot ask them for assistance." She added,

> If I was very sick, I know my daughters would come here and take care of me. But I am not sick that way [meaning a terminal diagnosis]. I have arthritis, and this will disable me. It is a long drawn out condition.

Nazi's medical condition confines her; it contributes to her isolation and loneliness. The question that arises is: Ultimately, should society not bear the responsibility for taking care of socially marginalized persons through its social and health institutions? In the context of this study, the persons in question are those who have been subject to structural exclusion after migrating to a new country, an exclusion that made the study participants feel that they were still displaced. They had lost the social milieu of their homeland, but it had not been replaced in Canada. Nazi and her cohort referred to having barely any Caucasian friends at a level where they could get together for coffee and chat. My re-reading of the transcript suggests that what Nazi desired was affirmation of life achieved through traces left for the living, a dimension that could form part of social palliation.

Goli: Can Palliative Care Accommodate the "Trauma" of Displacement and Re-Settlement?

Goli had the above question in mind when she suggested that I meet her at a North Shore senior housing complex. I was perplexed by her choice of location, as this was not where she lived. Arriving ten minutes early, I sat in the lounge on a torn sofa. It was not an inviting place; the people who moved in and out hardly exchanged words. Goli came ten minutes late, explaining that it took her time to walk from the bus stop to the complex. She wished to share her story from this place – a visceral undertaking. Below is a profile she mapped over two sessions: one in the lounge and one at a coffee shop. In addition, we conversed informally at her residence and during a walk on a nearby street. Speaking as a protagonist, Goli stated,

> When I first came to Canada with my husband Ahmed, we lived with our married daughter. She called us to look after her two children while she worked, not an atypical situation. Once the children started school, we decided to move out. The apartment was too small for all of us. We rented an apartment close by. But the rent kept on going up and up and up. We did not have an income and we did not want to take any money from our daughter. They have a young family. Once as I was walking on the street, tears flowed from my eyes. An Iranian woman approached me and asked me if she could help. I told her my financial problems. She gave me information on seniors' housing.

Goli put in an application. She said that this was not easy because initially no one helped her to fill out the forms, and it was very difficult for her to understand the requirements. It took time for Goli to discover that a seniors' committee was available to assist her in this task. She noted, "My English is good, but not that good." After one year, Goli learned that she and her husband had gotten a place – this was where I met her. Pointing to the complex, she said, first, "Look, the apartment they offered us is on the first floor. I am afraid of thieves. What will I do if someone breaks in?" Second, she noted that the apartment smelled of urine. "They refused to change the carpets. No one can live in a smelly place." Third, she pointed out that the apartment building was located on a hilly terrain away from bus stops, stores, and the doctor's office.

Goli stated, "My husband has arthritis. He will not be able to go out if we are not near a bus stop or stores." For all these reasons, Goli rejected the offer. She was informed that she had been placed on a wait list for another placement that would take over a year.

Moving into the senior housing complex would have compromised the couple's health because they would not have been able to go out, visit the doctor, or purchase vegetables and fruits from nearby stores. Staying in their present apartment and continuing to pay a high rent was the price that the couple had to pay to maintain their health for which purpose they engaged in self-care: eating healthy foods, going out for walks, and paying regular visits to the doctor. Goli gave two reasons. First, "In this country, we have to take care of our own health. Our children are busy. They will not be able to take care of us." Second, "not all medication is covered by the government. We do not have a lot of money, so we have to make sure that we remain healthy." Goli explained that they had sold their apartment in Iran and brought the money to Canada. Considering the conversion rate, this did not amount to much money. "We are living on our savings," she observed, and this was very stressful for her. She worried about what they would do if they ran out of money. She repeated that they would not ask their daughter as they knew that she and her family were struggling too.

When the subject matter of palliative care came up, Goli commented,

> You have explained to us the wonderful services that are offered to people who are dying. We get the food we like, and we are treated nicely. Should they not address our everyday stress that is causing us to fall sick or even die from it? What about financial issues? What about loneliness and isolation that we seniors experience every day of our lives?

Goli is quick to juxtapose the present and the past. Her remembrance of life in Iran is that of everyday social interactions. "You come out of the house and there is always someone to talk to, even if it comes down to saying '*salam*' (greeting meaning peace). I did not know what isolation was like until I came here." She added that in Iran, they owned their own house and Ahmed had a job. "He tried to find work here – any kind of work – but no one would hire him." She repeatedly stated, "We only came here to be close to our daughter. We cannot live in Iran without our children and grandchildren." Having heard about family-centred palliative care from a friend, she said, "I am filled with anxiety if my daughter has to take care of us. She is busy with work and family."

Goli understood that palliative care would provide material support to her or her husband if necessary. But she knew that the emotional burden of care would fall on her daughter. Knowing how hard her daughter worked, Goli had not shared the everyday problems that she was facing – the narrative of immigrant struggle (loneliness and having to take care of chores in their old age). When I asked her about her views on palliative care, she stated, "Rather than compassionate care, I would like social care and I would like them to learn about our struggles." She added, "Compassionate care at the time of death does not include our life situations. *The struggles of real life are wiped away if you are only nice to us when we are dying*" (my emphasis).

Goli's memorialization of her life story suggests that social palliation might look at pain and suffering caused not by illness, but by the trauma of displacement. Here, we may note that this trauma is brought about by structural factors. Left to fend for themselves, aging and older immigrants do not receive acknowledgement or validation of their experiences. One way in which social palliation could remedy this situation is to nurture a social milieu that does not individualize one's suffering. Goli raises two interrelated questions: Why does suffering need to be medicalized to receive attention? Does social suffering not matter? Her questions echo Das's (1997) observation that suffering may be "defined as an assemblage of human problems that have their origins and consequences in the devastating injuries that social forces inflict on human experience. *It is in collective life that individuals seek to understand their experiences and to work towards healing*" (571, emphasis added). Like other participants, Goli seeks to be part of a collective life that could constitute the layered landscape of social palliation.

To do justice to Goli's memorialization of life here (Canada) and there (Iran), I would like to present the experience of deep trauma (social wounding) that she and her peers are subject to. I argue that storied memory work is integral to articulating this trauma. My visits to Goli, particularly our walking trip on a street near Lonsdale, revealed that the place where she lived was not merely a geographical or physical space. She had reconstituted her immediate environment so that it carried traces of memories from Iran.

> See this place [an office], an Iranian realtor works there. He is looking for a low-rental place for us. He is very friendly. Sometimes when I feel down, I go and talk to him. I talk about my life in Iran. I think he likes talking to me because I give him news from Iran. And it makes him remember his own life there.

As we continue to walk, Goli chats with some Iranian women whom she has come to know gradually. This practice constitutes the everyday space of interactions. The encounter is brief – they exchange notes on health, illness, and their families – yet such exchanges are critically important, as Manderson and Allotey (2003) and Dyck and Dossa (2007) have noted. These spaces are critical to women's sense of belonging; their reference points include memories of home embedded in a world of relationships. Dyck (2017) notes that when women have the opportunity to form dense, dynamic networks (thickly lived places as opposed to thinly lived places), they tend to feel more at home as they learn more about how the host society differs from their life in their homeland. But this opportunity is not equally available to all. And the constituency for whom these spaces and places are least available is older immigrant women, who are not necessarily mobile or who do not have the resources to move around. But even for younger women (and men), the issue remains, because they do not have much time for daily social interactions. And their structural exclusion renders their situation more difficult because it leads to a divide between utilitarian work-based relationships and affect-based social relationships. It is ironic that the former relationships are time-consuming, yet offer minimal opportunities for enduring friendships (*doosti*) between established/white residents and newcomers/immigrants.

Moving into the social housing apartment would have diminished the small network of relationships that Goli had formed; this would have compromised her healing from the social wounds of having to struggle alone in a new place. While she struggles financially in her current apartment, remaining there at least allows her to maintain a social world. But this precariousness worries Goli; it is a burden (*mozahem*) that she carries like a wound. She stated,

> Not a day goes by when I don't think of what will happen when we run out of our savings? Our rent keeps on going up and up? What will happen if we are no longer able to pay the rent? Will our option be to go into the streets [*stated in a bitter tone*]?

A plea to be seen and heard arises from deeply felt suffering (the wound). It is this trauma that compels Goli to address palliative care practitioners with the message that "being nice to us when we are approaching the end-of-life is not enough. Consider our life stories and see what we have lost." What is remembered of a life left behind does not merely refer to a way of life that is lost, but to a vision that one seeks to rejuvenate in a new place. This vision is not abstract; it is critical for survival. If a story can take the form of recovery of the human voice, this occurs not at the level of utterance but in a form that might animate words and give them life, as Das (2015) states it.

Goli's frustration at her inability to rejuvenate life in a new place renders her a wounded storyteller. She is concerned that a time will come when she will be left alone in her apartment. She is not a stranger to this scenario. She observed,

> My life is not that different from other [Iranian] women of my age. They too came to this country to be near their children. They would not have come otherwise. We older people are better off in Iran but not without our families. When we come here, we find that our children are *very, very busy* (emphasis in the original). We cannot make any demands on them. Even financially, they are struggling. They have their own children that they must educate in a world that is very hard. My husband is not keeping well. One day, I will find myself alone. I am wondering if I cannot get up from my chair, who will be there to help me?

Not being able to get up from one's chair is a metaphor that aptly captures the life situation of an elderly immigrant woman. The ambiguity of her family being near yet not being there for her is not lost on Goli. Sitting on a sofa draped with Iranian embroidered cushions, she observed,

> My daughter takes me to doctor's appointments. She never refuses when I ask her. But I do not ask her too often. Sometimes when I am sick, and I can tolerate it, I tolerate it and hope that I will get well. I try some home remedies.

When I asked Goli to give me an example of a time when her daughter took her to the doctor, she said,

> I had a stomach ache that would not go away. My daughter took some time off work and took me to the doctor. She brought her phone [iPad], and I could see she had a lot of work to do. The doctor made us sit for an hour though he only saw me for ten minutes. My daughter dropped me off at home with some medication. That was it.

Goli's words, "that was it," suggest that there was not much discussion between her and her daughter about non-medical matters. This is because her daughter was in a hurry. This narrative is not unusual; other study participants shared similar stories.

Because Goli was finding it difficult to walk, I asked her if her daughter had investigated home-care services. Goli was already familiar with the services her husband was receiving for his care. But she dismissed this as peripheral compared with her greater need for social interactions.

In *Aging and the Indian Diaspora,* Lamb (2009) asks two questions: Who should care for elderly persons? And what is the best place for them to live: with family, alone, or in a seniors' home? Her questions are prompted by the forces of globalization that I have discussed in this book in the context of neoliberal global capitalism. We may note that this system entails the restructuring and devolution of the social service sector, accentuating the disadvantaged status of aging immigrants because of their structural exclusion in the host society. I would like to emphasize that neoliberalism does not merely consist of economic reforms. It is a system of governmentality underpinned by a moral order of self-interest and self-actualization as opposed to a socio-centric view of the world. This system of governance swallows the labour of younger members of the family while at the same time putting the onus on them to take care of their elderly kin. But the assumed family care is not in place. Khadija put it emphatically, "It is not that our family does not love us. They just do not have the time. They are too pressurized in this country. We cannot add to their pressures."

Goli's last words were, "Take care of my housing situation." Goli is seeking a place that would connect to the outside world of sociality; the system's notion of a house is that of a place of physical habitation. Fostering sociality, as I show through the pages of this book, forms an important component of social palliation.

Conclusion: Wounded Storytellers

In this chapter, I have shown that displacement as a critical life event continues in the country of settlement through structural exclusion, and is felt more intensely through the neoliberal regime that fosters individualism, self-care, and self-responsibility. These attributes have a generational effect, exacerbated for racialized minorities. While younger people are compelled to invest heavily in the neoliberal market sphere, aging persons are left to fend for themselves. Both cohorts feel trapped because they are not presented with alternatives. Fifty-five-year-old Farida explained, "In the workplace, they do not take into consideration that you might be caring for your aging parents. Work or quit: this is the message we receive." Eighty-five-year-old Kulsum put it this way,

If we do not encourage our children to work hard, how will they succeed in life? We must consider that they have their own children, family life, and pressurized work. We don't always tell them if we have problems.

My conversations with palliative care practitioners revealed an assumption that patients from racialized minority communities have access to family support. Yet the above observations illustrate a diminished support system, an issue that must not be taken lightly because it affects the conditions under which people experience life conjoined with death. Misunderstanding the situation, practitioners make room for families to spend time with their loved ones at the end of their lives. Under pressure that their loved ones will not live for long, families take on the "holistic work" of palliative care by providing physical, emotional, social, and spiritual support. If family members manage to get together, this is because they take time off work on compassionate grounds, or because they have travelled from other places. Overlooked here is the reality that before a person is admitted into palliative care, they may have spent considerable time being lonely and isolated. Indeed, such a situation was not unusual for older study participants. Loneliness and isolation are existential issues. They amount to losing one's connections to the world, creating a deep sense that one's life experiences, including one's understanding of how life ultimately gives way to death, are not shared with others. Storied lives bring into relief the point that death does not occur in isolation from lived realities. This ispoignantly brought home by wounds of displacement incurred through the geo-politics of border-crossings.

3 Precarity as a Resource for Life and Death

The theoretical concept of precarity is gaining ground across disciplinary boundaries. This concept draws our attention to the blurred boundary between the precariousness of life in the biological sense of the word and precarity that refers to structural and socio-cultural barriers exacerbating one's social marginality (Butler 1997, 2012; Shaw 2018).[1] Of interest is the fact that the social condition of precarity does not allow one to fall out of life. In fact, it can be used as a resource for living and dying because this trajectory takes shape in the form of a relationship between a person and the world. It is in this context that anthropologist Hayder Al-Mohammad (2016) identifies the dynamic whereby we can fall out of the world but also belong to it. When worlds break down, he argues, they open spaces to explore how social life may be sustained. He notes that "inquiries into medicine and ill health have done much to make precarious the grip personhood has on well-being, worldhood and life itself and to indicate some of the possible tensions or frailties inherent in being-in-the-world" (465). Precarity is of interest as it "can foster not just the degradation of life but the imagined capacity to redefine the existential meaning of present conditions" (Shaw 2018, 41).

My goal in this chapter is to show how precarity, with its tenuous hold on life, can be used as a resource for living and dying. It could also be a resource for social palliation whereby one can draw on emotional, social, and aesthetic support in the context of reciprocal relationships that are fostered organically in everyday life. This focus enables us to remain "attentive to the enormous efforts made by ordinary people to provide space of affirmation, joy and care through a kind of ordinary realism about life and death" (Fassin 2016, 771). Holding on to the possibility of life folded into death requires close attention to the analytic of everyday life. Following Das (2007), I argue that life is rejuvenated through a descent into the ordinary.[2] As Garcia (2016) has observed, everyday routines of life "are produced at the intersection of individual agency and social constraints" (322). It is in this context that I explore how suffering and the uncertainty of life can open different horizons of meaning, existing between being-in-the-world and falling out of it. To illustrate, I present a reading of four singular lives: (a) Mirza, a Baha'i who migrated to Canada with his son, daughter, and wife to escape intense persecution in his home country of Iran; (b) Rubina, an Ismaili-Muslim who left Kenya with her husband and son because of economic precarity; (c) Shabina, who migrated to Canada from Iran in search of care for her differently abled son; and (d) Mobina, whose migration was prompted by the economic exclusion of Ismailis/Asians in Kenya. Acting as protagonists, they narrate their life stories from particular social locations. My focus on singular life narratives is meant to communicate the depth of my participants' experiences and to "illuminate the complex intimate and structural relations that constitute a life, a community, and a social world" (Garcia 2010, 72). Their singular narratives are bound up with others, a point echoed by Frank: "Storytelling is for another just as much as it is for oneself" (1995, 18).

All of them came to Canada in the eighties. My analysis of the content of the narratives relayed at multiple sites (homes, streets, hospitals, and cafeterias) is informed by the narrators' attempts to simultaneously hold onto life while being aware that they can fall out of it as they confront the trajectory of life and death. I ask two key questions raised by Das and Han (2016): "How might we attend to the fragility of life in the sense of a human form of life?" and "How is death absorbed within life?" (17). Study participants' responses to these questions are embedded in border-crossing stories on life and death.

Mirza: Escaping Persecution

"There was a revolution in Iran of the kind that cannot be reversed. Every part of the country was affected. Our education system was changed overnight to reflect its Islamic character. It is now 'The Islamic Republic of Iran,'" mused Amir, an Iranian, during a conversation at a dinner party. Mirza's experience was more intense.

> When the revolution occurred, we Bahai's had a very hard time. They gave us the message that we were not wanted in Iran. If we touched the fruit in a produce store, we were told off. The government would not give us jobs. Some of my friends were killed.

The persecution of the Bahai's touched their very sense of being-in-the-world. It was this aspect that prompted Mirza and his family to leave "his beloved country," his home embedded in memories of growing up and building a life despite long-standing persecution that waxed and waned. Consider the following excerpt from the Baha'i International Community (https://www.bic.org/):

> Since the Islamic Revolution, the Baha'is have been systematically perse-cuted as a matter of government policy. During the first decade of this per-secution, more than 200 Baha'is were killed or executed, hundreds more were tortured or imprisoned, and tens of thousands lost jobs, access to education, and other rights – all solely because of their religious belief. Government-led attacks on the country's largest non-Muslim religious minority have re-intensified in the last decade. Since 2005, more than 820 Baha'is have been arrested, and the number of Baha'is in prison has risen from fewer than five to more than 80. The list of prisoners includes all seven members of a former leadership group serving the Baha'i commu-nity of Iran. In 2010, the seven were wrongly sentenced to twenty years in prison, the longest term currently facing any prisoner of conscience in Iran. Recent reports indicate that their sentences have been reduced from twenty years to ten years, in line with changes to the Iranian Penal Code introduced in May 2013. The constant threat of raids, arrests, and deten-tion or imprisonment is among the main features of Iran's persecution of Baha'is today.

Warin and Dennis (2008) have this to say:

> Since its inception in the 19th century, followers of the Baha'i faith have been persecuted for their "heretic" beliefs and have been subject to exclu-sion, imprisonment and execution (most notably – by the Shah's secret police – the SAVAK). It was, however, during, and after the Islamic Revo-lution of 1979 and the installing of the tighter Islamic laws that the Baha'is experienced new levels of overt discrimination and violence. (103; also see Momen 2012, Yazdani 2012)

Mirza had no choice but to leave Iran with his family in the mid-1980s. He was drawn to Canada because of its global image of humanitarian-ism and peace. His desire was to settle down and live a life of dignity that had been denied to him, his family, and his compatriots in their homeland. He specified two primary goals: to secure a livelihood, criti-cal for one's well-being, and to seek a good life for his differently abled son. As I got to know Mirza, I realized that, ultimately, he was seeking (not unlike other study participants) to convey the message that life could not be lived without an understanding of its intricate connection to death. And death would be devoid of meaning if it did not continue to inform the lives of the living. People who have been subject to suffering and precarity have a keen understanding of this existential issue. My analytical understanding of this matter is that one does not simply fall out of life.

Mirza's Life Narrative: "In Iran, I was part of a persecuted community. In Canada, my family and I were left alone to fend for ourselves"

Mirza and his wife Juliet have a son named Alfred who is forty-two years old, and, as Mirza noted, has the IQ of a fourteen-year-old boy. They, and their daughter, came to Canada as refugees fleeing religious persecution, noted above. What kind of persecution did Mirza and his family experience in Iran? And what are the conditions under which they were left to fend for themselves in Canada? In response to these questions, Mirza tells an intertwined story, connecting "here" (Canada) and "there" (Iran) by taking us, the readers, to scenarios of his life in both countries. This connection reveals his position of simultaneously being-in-the-world and falling out of it, along with his engagement in re-making a world across multiple borders. On a broader level, Mirza's socio-cultural connection between "here" and "there" reflects the hitherto unarticulated connection between the global North and the global South. As I have argued elsewhere (Dossa 2014), we must recognize the significance of this connection if we are to write a different kind of story.

Iranian Tea in Transparent Glasses/Canadian Coffee in White Mugs

My meetings with Iranian participants in their homes did not take place without the serving of Iranian tea in transparent glasses, complemented with cubes of sugar, and nuts arranged aesthetically on a tray. I considered this to be a gesture of hospitality, which I experienced during my brief visits to Iran (1994 and 2003). Mirza drew a comparison between Iranian tea and Canadian coffee, not in relation to taste or preference, but symbolically. For him, the image of Iranian tea represents sociality; it is shared with kith and kin. The Canadian mug of coffee represents a more limited sociality: meeting one friend or colleague for a chat. Mirza's comparison was meant to serve a larger point, namely his isolation in the country of settlement – an isolation that is compounded by the "trauma" that he (the protagonist of his story) experienced before he migrated. This isolation is captured in his reflection that Iranian tea (or food) is prepared for many people, not for one person, like the Canadian mug of coffee. To make sense of his suffering over "there" (Iran) and over "here" (Canada), Mirza connects the two countries through sensual experience, a connection sustained in his account.

Mirza relayed the historical persecution of his community and how this affected his life and that of his family. This persecution formed part of everyday life in Iran: he treaded a rocky path to obtain his education as an accountant yet was not hired despite his qualifications. He was sent to a small place by the government and given the job of a "delivery man," which he struggled to retain as he was the only breadwinner in his family. Eventually, he was hired by a bank, but he was fired from this job after a few years, along with other Baha'is. A pension was promised to him, but it stopped after six months.

Realizing that he did not have any prospects in Iran, he made the decision to emigrate. He chose Canada over United States because Canada allows new residents to visit their homeland after a period of six months. Such was his attachment to Iran, a country he refers to as his "dear homeland," despite the long-standing exclusion of his community from citizenship rights. Unfortunately, the promise of a return visit did not materialize: the cost of airfare was prohibitive.

Mirza cannot afford a car. Where he lives, there are no stores except for a corner grocery, and so he uses public transit for shopping and everyday chores. While he seems to have accepted this way of life – going everywhere by transit– he finds it especially difficult when it comes to taking his son to a family doctor. Without access to a car, these regular visits are arduous. By means of enactment (bodily expressions), Mirza described these trips, stating,

> It takes one and a half hours to transit to the clinic in Vancouver by bus. We are made to wait for the doctor. Sometimes it takes as long as two hours. It takes me an entire day to visit a doctor for my son. And this in a situation where the doctor spends ten to fifteen minutes with us.

Through his son's medical visits, Mirza came to realize that his expectations of life in Canada would remain unrealized. He had hoped that a new and supposedly welcoming country would help his family to heal. His impression of Canada was that of a place where he could build a dignified life for himself and his son. But in addition to losing almost an entire day in transit, he finds that commuting and waiting for long hours do not contribute to his son's well-being. The discrepancy

of spending so much time commuting only to receive minimal attention from the doctor reveals the intense marginalization experienced by
Mirza and his son. This discrepancy further reveals the fault lines of a
system that assumes a person's time is of no value, a system that keeps
a person waiting. This system does not recognize Mirza and his son as
people who are struggling to settle down in a new country. When one
remains unnoticed by society, especially by a system from which one
expects compassion, it compromises one's sense of being-in-the-world.
At work here is cloak time, which Stevenson (2014) refers to as "anonymous care" that she defines as being "indifferent to who precisely is
being cared for, thus in some sense standardizing what it means to care"
(163). In this context, she argues that caring is subject to measurement
and evaluation, devoid of emotional qualities. The underlying theme is
that there are other ways of being in time that Mirza and his family do
not experience owing to their intense isolation in Canada.

In Iran, Mirza was subject to prejudice and exclusion that were overt,
in the open. In Canada, he feels excluded in ways that he cannot name,
except through particular experiences. He noted that he barely knows
his neighbours:

> We do not exchange greetings. They [Canadians of European origin] think
> that we are from another planet. They avoid us in different ways like
> sometimes not riding on the elevator with us or pretending that we are
> just not there.

For Mirza and his family, this experience is painful. His neighbours are
aware that he is a newcomer, yet they have not inquired as to who he is,
or how he and his family have settled in. This form of isolation deserves
attention in a society where relationships of "neighbours-as-strangers"
are normalized and barely questioned. Consider what Phelps (2004) has
to say:

> Even as we narrate our individual stories, these stories we tell about our-
> selves and our lives are not autonomous, disconnected units. As we shape
> the discordant events of our lives into a coherent narrative, we also dis-
> cover our "place" in larger units in our families, communities, and nations.
> *Our identity depends on our place in relation to others and to our community.*
> (58, emphasis added)

Mirza's story of isolation speaks to a loss of proximity, to use Han's
(2016) term. Proximity refers to situations where one can engage in
conversation with another person on the street, or in a neighbourhood.

Mirza remarks that there are people around him – neighbours, pass-ersby, shoppers – but that he does not really know them. As a member of a religious minority, he feels that he does not quite belong to the Iranian community concentrated on the North Shore, which in any case is quite a distance from his residence in Coquitlam. Mirza's loss of social milieu translates into the loss of a social world. The inability to foster a relational identity constitutes a wound, one from which a story is likely to emanate. Between seeking to recover his lost social world and realizing that isolation is part of the way of life that his country of settlement offers, Mirza occupies a liminal space between being-in-the-world and falling out of it. He left Iran to forestall the possibility of falling out of the world and now finds himself in this delicate balance. His position of falling, almost, out of the world comes across in his exposition, offered below, of how his son's health and well-being was compromised in their homeland.

Securing Everyday and Life

Mirza and Juliet are preoccupied with the care of their son, Alfred. When he was young, Alfred's health was affected by an episode of high fever, from which he recovered. Mirza stated,

> After that initial episode, he was extremely healthy, and went to school on time like the other children. He appeared to be a normal boy who was curious, outgoing, and confident. In grade three there were some children who bullied him.

The bullying Alfred experienced was not addressed by the school. It continued, and led to a major incident that Mirza described as follows:

> There was a religious event for Muslims on a Friday night. Even though this wasn't a school night, most students were attending this event held at the school. Alfred didn't want to attend because we are Baha'i. The religious day was not of importance to us and therefore we didn't force him to attend. At the end of the school day, the principal, knowing that he was not attending, took him to the basement of the school and hit him hard on the head. It was not unusual for teachers or principals to hit their students if they disagreed with their instructions. After this incident, we saw a change in his personality and behaviour. He became a very angry boy. He would have frequent bursts of anger all the while feeling very nervous and anxious. His confidence plummeted, and he was always scared, even to go to the washroom alone. He stopped talking, but instead would keep

his opinions and thoughts to himself. He used to be an intelligent, courageous, and confident boy, but quickly turned shy and easily frightened.
After seeing this dramatic change in personality, we took him to see a
psychiatrist. He was given medication to control his mood. His condition
progressed and became much worse. We took him to see many different
specialists, and he had a CT scan as well as an MRI that didn't show anything unusual. He was constantly trying different medications to control
his anxiety, his nervousness, and most seriously his seizures. Because of
his progressing mental condition, he developed a learning disability, and
it was difficult for him to comprehend and retain information. He only
finished up to grade eleven.

Mirza has a purpose in recalling a past event in his home country. For
him, the past is present, embodying and encompassing his son's life.
And it is his son's differently abled body that establishes the connection
between "there" and "here." Mirza bemoans the fact that over "here,"
his son has not had the opportunity to heal. The family has been left
to its "own meagre resources" to make the best of their situation. Yet,
Mirza takes up the challenge of being-in-the-world, of not falling out
of it. He does this by securing everyday life for Alfred. Das (2003) notes
that it is on the register of everyday life that we can document a double
movement: at the macro-level of the political system and at the micro-
level of families and communities:

> The self-creation on the register of the everyday is a careful putting
> together of life – a concrete engagement with the tasks of remaking that
> is mindful of the compounded expression – everyday and life. It points to
> the "eventedness of the everyday" and the attempt to forge oneself into an
> ethical subject within this scene of the ordinary. (302)

Mirza's Baha'i status made it relatively easy for him to enter Canada.
As a persecuted community, the Baha'is were given preference. Once he
and his family arrived in Canada, however, they were left on their own.
Other than cursory and pamphlet-based information about services in
Canada, no assistance was given to Mirza to help him and his family
feel at home in a new place, and, more important, to help him secure a
job. One person was assigned to help the family settle in, but this person
was constantly out of town. The family received government funding
for one year, after which Mirza was compelled to go on welfare.

Lest we think that this situation is unusual, consider Rahder and
McLean's (2013) work on newcomers in Toronto, Canada. Observing
the expansive reach of neoliberalism, they contend that this regime of

power has continuously eroded public spaces and service infrastructure. This erosion structurally disenfranchises people on the margins of society.

Mirza and his wife devote their time to caring for their son – a responsibility that they have taken on earnestly because they have no other social support. Reflecting on this lack, Mirza recalled everyday life in his homeland:

> In Iran, all the relatives would drop in, and they would take Alfred out. Since we moved here, he does not have the family support that he once had. In Iran, he had more family members who would visit and talk to him and take him around town and out of the house. *Here he's stuck indoors most of the time and does not have the opportunity to socialize* [*stated in a low voice with much sadness*].

Pointing to the bags of groceries that he carried home on the bus, Mirza observed, "Back home, everything was close by. We did not have to travel long distances to get to a store." In Iran, Mirza was emplaced in the sense that his excursions for work or shopping entailed social interactions. Other study participants reiterated this point, remembering the neighbourhoods of their homeland as social spaces where there were always people with whom they could have a conversation. Social interactions occurred whenever they left the house, even if this was in the simple form of *salam* (peace greeting) followed by an inquiry about one's family's well-being. For Mirza, the isolation of being confined to the house without the opportunity for social interaction is as painful as a wound on one's body. However, he understands the family must survive, socially and otherwise, which means striving to remain part of the world rather than falling out of it. It is in this context that Mirza has encouraged his son to cultivate a daily routine:

> He wakes up at around 6:30 a.m. and does his morning prayer, and then afterwards, if no one is awake, he will go back to sleep. He usually gets out of bed around 8:00 to 9:00 a.m. and does some light exercises, such as stretching for five to ten minutes. He likes to sleep, and it is usually with great trouble that we get him out of bed. He eats six to seven times a day and uses the washroom three times a day for an hour at a time. When he's asked, he will do some chores like wash the dishes or sweep, but he won't do it on his own. We remind him to do something a couple of times before he responds and carries out the task, because his brain doesn't process the information quickly. He walks around the house to pass time or sometimes walks to the convenient store down the street to get a food item. But he

has low energy and gets tired quickly when he walks or does something. He doesn't leave the house very much because he needs assistance. He also can get very obsessive about certain things, especially about doing a certain task at hand. For example, if I ask him to sweep the kitchen, he will spend a long time sweeping, and then sweeping again, and again, before he stops. Also, he doesn't talk very much, unless we direct a question to him. In that case he will answer, but he won't elaborate on his answers. Oftentimes when he gets angry, he will hit his head with his hands. He usually sleeps around 11:00 p.m.

On the surface, Alfred's confinement to the domestic sphere can be attributed to his medical condition. But a closer reading reveals a macro-level scenario whereby Alfred's life is restricted by the lack of social services and vocational training that are in place for people with disabilities, albeit unequally and hierarchically based on one's race, gender, and class (Dossa 2009). The unavailability of services reflects Mirza's displacement in Canada: his lack of fluency in English has prevented him from seeking assistance, and no one has reached out to help him. There is also a complex factor at work. Mirza wishes his son could have a life in which he is cared for as a person, and not as a client, as someone who is "disabled." He does not wish his son's care to be part of the competitive, individualistic, and market-oriented value system prevalent in the host society. Mirza does not think that such a system would meet his son's need for sociality.

In light of the above situation, Mirza and his wife have little choice but to ensure their son's well-being to the extent possible. To maintain stability, they assign him mundane tasks such as sweeping floors, or encourage him to pick up items from the nearby convenience store. This is his outing. In Iran, Alfred had a job that had been given to him by a relative. It kept him occupied and gave him a sense of satisfaction. In Canada, being confined to the home is difficult for Alfred. There is no meaningful change of scenery. Apart from the arduous journeys to the doctor's office, the convenience store is his only regular contact with the outside world.

Considering how Alfred's everyday life unfolds in time and space, an uncritical reading would suggest that it is his ill health that keeps him confined to the domestic sphere. However, this confinement is compounded by other factors, for instance the language barrier that he and his parents face. Language can be learned in many ways, formal and informal, but the family has been short-changed on both counts. Formally, they have not been introduced to ESL programs in a sustained way. Informally, their opportunities to acquire fluency through everyday interactions with neighbours are highly limited by the "gated community" structure of their neighbourhood, in which enclosures diminish the possibility for social interactions (Low 2004).

Yet, in the wake of these compounded limitations, Alfred cultivates small spaces in the context of his everyday life. While small, the importance of these spaces cannot be dismissed; there are no grand projects of recovery. As Das had pointed out, "One could occupy the space of devastation by making it one's own not through a gesture of escape but by occupying it in its present-ness" (2003, 299). The issue becomes one of undertaking everyday tasks that make social survival possible. Alfred's daily routine, his morning prayers and exercise, his tasks around the house, impart some meaning to his life. They give him something to do. A trip to the convenience store, however brief, provides him with a sense of engagement with the outside world. He dresses up for this trip as if for an outing, and his regular visits lead to small talk with the store owner. These small events allow him to assume a subject position, even though it is not free from the social wound that he and his family incur from the lack of human proximity.

Act of Witnessing

As I came to know Mirza through his words, and through his gentle, soft-spoken manner, I realized that his storied account constitutes an act of witnessing with a twofold goal. First, the act of witnessing requires one to assume the position of a subject. Through this subjectivity, which emerges out of the experience of being subjugated, one can engage with the body politic, unsettling and interrogating taken-for-granted aspects of reality. The second goal of witnessing calls attention to the way in which the personal and political are intertwined. In his account, Mirza indicated that he is aware of the multiple ways in which his intimate life is affected by structures of power. It is in this vein that he shares his wife's experience of pain and suffering:

> After we arrived, my wife had a medical emergency. The vein in her leg stiffened. We had to rush her to the hospital because she was in excruciating pain (*dard*). The hospital gave her morphine to help with the pain while she was waiting in the emergency ward. We were waiting three to five hours before seeing a physician. The physician gave her more morphine and prescribed her ten to fifteen sessions of physiotherapy and massages. We believe that her pain is stress induced. She has been very upset

and worried about her daughter's husband, who is abusive, as well as our son who has a medical condition. She goes into states of depression (*afsordegi*).

Mirza's account is reminiscent of Nancy Scheper-Hughes's (1992) observation that the hungry are medicated rather than fed. Structural factors are masked in such a situation, and so they remain unaddressed. Here, we have an example of what Das refers to as a kind of "suffering which takes us from the social to the individual body written within the framework of political economy" (1997, 566). Such situations, she argues, should give us "the ability to think otherwise" (2016, 168). My analysis of Mirza's position as witness suggests that he wishes to communicate the politics of exclusion through the avenue of his lived reality, even as he undertakes this task with a sense of gentleness, as is his demeanour. But more than this, he seeks to tell a larger story for humanity, a term that he uses often and that he co-opts to transform his experiences into a case "for everyone, not for myself only."

Mirza is aware of the contradiction of his refugee status in Canada. His acceptance into the country does not extend beyond the minimal act of admission. He says that he appreciates the "safety and freedom" that Canada offers, and he embraces the country's multicultural milieu, in which he hopes to find a niche. "Naturally, we feel comfortable walking around on the streets." But his everyday experiences reveal more subtle discomforts that dilute his initial impressions of life in a new place. He observes that Canada's multiculturalism does not offer much depth beyond the notion that people of different cultural backgrounds might live together. He notes that accomplishing basic errands is made difficult by the lack of nearby stores, requiring him to travel long distances by transit to purchase groceries. "I do not have a car as I cannot afford one." His monthly rent is $1,300, and another $135 is spent on cable, internet, and telephone. None of the family members are in the workforce; with these expenses, they barely survive on welfare. The contradiction of Mirza's life in Canada is that various barriers – unemployment, long commutes, inaccessible places, and language barriers – accumulate to produce a situation in which he feels cut off and alone. "When we first arrived, everything was new for us and we liked everything. However, more and more we are feeling isolated and lonely." It was not difficult for me to map the family's isolation from its surroundings. There are very few places for social interaction, let alone for fostering sustained relationships where they live.

Mirza challenges us to make sense of the human experience of isolation and loneliness. It is in this context that he acts as a witness to his own story, suggesting that it is morally wrong to live in a social world where human contact is so limited that we do not even acknowledge the presence of the people around us. His experience unsettles our normalized acceptance of gated communities and the lack of social interactions that they could generate. Mirza has inspired me to share my personal experience.

On one occasion, I was accidently locked out of my house without access to a phone. It was freezing cold and raining heavily. Using the cell phone of a passerby, I managed to get in touch with a locksmith. The locksmith did not show up within the promised time period of twenty minutes; I had to call him several more times, and had to ask my neighbours for assistance. I had come to know my neighbours "quite well" during my regular walks over the last fifteen years. But I found that meeting on the streets was one thing; knocking on their doors was quite a different experience. While the neighbours obliged and allowed me to use their phones, their act of assistance was carried out on the borderland, that is, the porch. I was not to cross the boundary that would allow me to enter their homes. Even though it was freezing cold and raining, the neighbours with whom I had chatted on the street over the years did not invite me into their homes. Through this experience, I realized how abnormal it was to live in a world where neighbours are largely strangers (not overlooking exceptions). Insecurity and fear of the Other trump ethical values of kindness and concern. We live in a world where we accept *socially empty spaces*.

Living and Dying

The act of witnessing is enabling. It effects a movement from the private to the public sphere, illustrating how a personal story is interwoven with the body politic. Such a movement can take us to the edge, the very frontier of death-in-life and life-in-death, as Das and Han (2016) would state it. Having depicted the events of his life, Mirza positioned himself to relay a larger story of living and dying. He is not afraid of death. He emphasizes that death should be considered part of life, not separate from it. He feels that he has lived his life, in the sense that things are not going to change for him. And although life has not been kind to Mirza, he chooses not to resign himself to its unkindness. Knowing that my research was concerned with palliative care, Mirza offered his perspective on care:

> I think a universal approach needs to be taken. It is important to remember that the person you're caring for is a mother, a sister, or a daughter. Staff

should remember to be kind to their patients and to give their patients a sense of hope. By being careful with the vocabulary that they use, they can avoid shattering the hope that their patients have. Patients need a companion in the hospital to talk to, and to listen to their beliefs. Hospital personnel don't have much time to provide emotional support, but patients are in great need of this type of care.

Mirza foregrounds two important questions: How can we give hope to the patient or the person receiving care? And how can we provide companionship that patients desire? As Mirza put it, "*Hospital personnel don't have much time to provide emotional support, but patients are in great need of this type of care*" (emphasis in the original). Mirza's reference to the hospital is in connection with his perspective on the larger issue of a caring society/social palliation. The provision of care is an exceedingly complex issue. While palliative care practitioners recognize the importance of social and emotional care, these values are not built into the system. Staff are busy with other things. My visits to hospices, hospitals, and nursing homes leave me with an image of hurried staff pushing carts in and out of residents' rooms – carts of laundry, of medication, and of meals. They are occupied with work that has more to do with the body than with affect. The importance of companionship becomes neglected in the medicalized focus on bed-and-body work (medication and comfort care). This gap is filled by family visits, and by a large body of volunteers who act as companions in palliative care facilities, and whose role is expressed metaphorically as "holding your hand."

Mirza's emphasis on the importance of emotional support in life and death echoes Lambek's (2016) question, "What is it that dies in the event of death and what is it that lives?" (625). Mirza provides an illuminating example:

I have held onto many pictures and memories over the years. In particular, I look back at my mother's picture and remember my childhood and the joys that ignorance brought. Being carefree and worry-free are times that I greatly miss. There's one picture of my mother, and I'm running in the back yard of our home, and she's chasing after me. In that moment things were so much simpler, and I didn't know the type of life that I would have ahead of me.

Mirza would say that the above passage has a "universal" appeal. To over-interpret this passage would not do justice to what the reader could take from it unmediated. Mirza invokes a scene from his childhood not merely to remember his mother – a powerful image on its own – but to convey the burden of life that he carries, the way he almost falls out of life.

Later, Mirza shares poems that he has written, and states that he wants to be remembered for his poetry and his words. "I want to be remembered by my intellect and ability to reason." A desire such as this is a far cry from the considerations of the medical system, which focuses its attention on the disease-ridden body, and has little room for active living (death-in-life). It is from this position of strength that Mirza considers the kind of care he would like for his son. He feels that he has lived his life, and now the focus should be on his son's life. Moreover, he worries about what will happen to his son's care when he and his wife are no longer around. He would like health professionals to care for his son in the community, and to ensure that he has part-time work where his condition of being differently abled is given consideration. Mirza knows that people with "disabilities" are not easily employed, but he also knows that "it is through work that my son will find happiness." He feels wounded that his son does not enjoy a better life in Canada, as he had envisioned.

Alfred did not participate in the research project. Hearing his father talk about death as integral to life – that we all have to die, but that the more important matter is what we have reaped from life and what opportunities life has given us – he stated, "I would want lots of people at my funeral. After I die, I would like lots of people to visit my grave." Evidently, Alfred is missing the world of social relationships that he enjoyed in his home country. Life and death are intertwined: without meaningful social interactions, we cannot reap from life so as to continue living after we have died (life-in-death). A full understanding and experience of death is derived from a world of sociality, from the interactions that occur as one goes about living a life.

Anthropologists have long argued for the significance of the ordinary and the everyday, because it is ultimately within these spaces, within the thinness or fullness of social relationships, that issues of living and dying unfold. Mirza experiences his greatest loss in the space of the everyday: he has lost the opportunity to live socially, and to provide a social life for his son. Sociality is a foundational component of life whose loss can amount to falling out of life. But this is not invariably the case. Al-Mohammad puts it this way, "Being-in-the world is as much about our ability to maintain a grip on the social meshwork as it is about our slipping and disentangling" (2016, 473). Mirza's life is lived between the spaces of being-in-the world and falling out of it. This liminality brings to light existential questions as to how we inhabit a world.

I present Mirza's life narrative not merely so that we might know his story, but for the broader purpose of acknowledging his life in the context of other lives. Mirza's singular story is part of the story of other displaced people who are making new lives for themselves in the West, where they are differentially valued and Othered. Beyond this, Mirza's life, his enmeshment between being-in-the-world and falling out of it, reveals the fragility and finitude of life. This fragility needs to be foregrounded in the contemporary world, where the loss of our bearings is most poignantly revealed in life's severance from death, and death's severance from life.

Rubina: "My grandson learnt to be compassionate watching how his grandfather was cared for by the family"

Seventy-six-year-old Rubina came to know of my project through word of mouth. She offered to share her story as she felt that there were unresolved issues in the death of her husband. Also, she had a good understanding of the impact of stories. "When we share our stories of *dukh* (sadness) and *sukh* (happiness), other people can learn from them. After all, it is through stories that we can connect with other people. Stories 'speak' and therefore they are touching." During our first meeting, she relayed the following incident.

> One day in Jamat Khana my grandson saw an older person stagger. To him, that man did not look well. He quickly found his father [Rubina's son] and told him there was a man who did not look well. "Come quickly, he told his father." So, my son and grandson rushed to that person and asked him how he was feeling. Realizing that he was critical, they contacted a First Aid Ismaili volunteer who called for an ambulance and the man was rushed to the hospital. Three weeks later this person passed away.

My reading of Rubina's narrative suggests her commitment to foreground the ethics of care sustained through being-in-the-world. She feels that the health/palliative care system failed her husband and that her experiential knowledge must not go to waste; it should be used to mitigate and heal other people's wounds. This is the angle that informed her telling of the story.

> You know, I want other people to benefit from my experiences. We should not have had to go through the struggles that we experienced while seeking care for my husband. As it is, when a person is sick, he/she is going through a lot. The system does not have to make it worse.

Rubina's point of entry into the ethics of care is her grandson: "It is amazing how this young child absorbed such compassion by observing what was happening to his sick grandfather." Her act of remembering her husband Navroz through her grandson is significant. It means that his life did not come to an end upon death; it became part of posterity, to be recalled and remembered contextually.

In remembering how her husband became sick and the series of events that ended in his death, Rubina highlights the attribute of compassion. This is how she remembers. Her memory work includes what is referred to as the immigrant story: the struggle to settle in a new place following displacement. Contrary to conventional understandings, this struggle goes beyond the issues of livelihood and shelter. It concerns rebuilding lives following the loss of a familiar environment, the rhythm of everyday life, and the network of relationships. What is lost is a milieu where one is recognized as a person as opposed to a racialized immigrant. In other words, the immigrant story concerns acquiring a sense of belonging to the world rather than falling out of it. It is in this context that Rubina observed,

> Navroz found it difficult to settle down. He was unhappy and depressed. He missed his Kenyan lifestyle. He missed his circle of friends. He wanted to return to Kenya. Life in Canada did not give him satisfaction. He wanted to go back but our children were well settled, and he did not want to uproot them.

Rubina is referring to a scenario that was repeatedly reiterated by other participants: "Over there in our home country we knew people. We engaged in relationships. This is why we miss our home. In Canada, you cannot interact with people. Either they are busy, or they are not interested in your life."

Navroz was caught between two worlds. According to Rubina, he could not settle down in Canada. "He wanted to go back to Kenya. He missed his friends and he missed his lifestyle." She added, "In Canada, it was just work. We had our own business and he had to work very hard to get this business off the ground. He only saw a life of work in Canada." In other words, he did not see a milieu of affect that would give him a sense of belonging to the world. Navroz could not go back to Kenya because his children were settling down well in Canada. "There were no opportunities in Kenya for education or careers. We did not want our two children (a girl and a boy) to come here on their own." This observation about the lack of opportunities in the home country requires a comment. Their home country was colonized by Britain.

Critical scholarship has highlighted the fact that colonization and neo-colonization has meant depletion of the resources and human power of the countries in question, which Allison (2013) refers to as the "New Scramble for Africa." These enterprises are not carried out in a vacuum. They entail undermining the ways of life of indigenous people, subjecting them to external control and governance. We live in a divided world, as the boundary between the global North and the global South, the First World and the Third World, is sharply drawn. This division affects our sense of well-being in our ability to be part of the world in which we live.

In the context of (neo)colonization, Navroz and his family's displacement can be understood as coercion: they were left with no other choice. According to Rubina, "our children's future comes first"; also, the Navrozes could not easily obtain a trade license for this business because of the policy of Africanization. Although Rubina did not make an explicit reference to racism, it would not be an exaggeration to state that Navroz felt excluded, an aspect that came to light when he became sick, and was also evident in his frequent returns to Kenya. In *Death and the Migrant*, Gunaratnam (2013) catches the sentiment that Navroz may have felt: "Some racisms you can know and name for what they are. Others are more slippery and shape-shifting, wriggling in and out of substance and language, intermingling and dissolving into other energies and currents" (48). It seems that Navroz lived on the borderland, his livelihood tied to Canada and his social relationships anchored in Kenya. Also, it must be kept in mind that the host environment's focus on integration makes it difficult for the immigrant generation to foreground and sustain their values, traditions, and practices integral to their sense of belonging to the world. Navroz's tenuous position of living between two worlds came to an end when he had a stroke that left him paralyzed. Rubina observed, "He would not have had a stroke. He was sent home a couple of times from the hospital with the message that he was alright. He was not *alright*" (emphasis in the original).

As Navroz's condition became worse, family members stepped in to take care of him. Rubina remained the primary caregiver while Navroz's sister and his son assisted. At one point, during heart surgery, he went into a coma. The cardiologist recommended that he be taken off life support. His son refused, stating, "Only God knows." Rubina had *satado* for Navroz, an Ismaili ritual whereby the whole congregation offers prayers in the Jamat Khana for seven days. "Nothing happened for six days. On the seventh day, my husband became conscious." He was then placed in a palliative room in the hospital. The circle of family members taking care of Navroz widened. All his sisters as well as

Rubina's sisters took turns visiting him. Meanwhile, a physiotherapist and a speech therapist helped him to recover. Rubina observed that his recovery was also facilitated by the fact that their daughter put family pictures on the wall and brought some tapes containing *ginans* and his favourite Bollywood songs. Navroz went home and was fine for a while. He even took a trip with his son to his homeland in Kenya.

Upon his return, he had another massive stroke. This time he was cared for from home. Rubina hired a young Filipino woman, Delya, to help take care of him, while his physio and speech therapy continued. Eventually, he regained his speech. Rubina attributed this to one additional factor: Delya had a young child who would sit on his lap and ask him to read her a story. Rubina noted, "His speech got better. We could not tell any difference from before."

Rubina was under a lot of stress. In her words, "Worrying about Navroz, sleepless nights, worrying about the children, emotional and physical stress, exhaustion physical and mental, lots of body aches and pains." She was resilient and felt that she had to be strong. She attended Jamat Khana early in the morning (4 a.m.), went for walks, and practised yoga. Eventually, she gave up her job with an advertising agency and stayed home. Equally healing was seeing her grandson "learn about the compassionate care that the family provided to my husband."

As Navroz's condition grew worse, he was admitted to a nursing home, not a hospice, as the family would have preferred. Realizing that the condition at the nursing home was not ideal, the family took on the responsibility of caring for him. They showered him, took him for walks, prepared his meals, and fed him. As Biehl (2005) has noted, in today's world, the family has increasingly become "the medical agent of the state" (22). Navroz collapsed again and was then given a palliative room in the hospital. After a few days, he ordered chai and cookies for the whole family. "It was a good day. He did not appear to be in any pain or discomfort. This was Saturday. On Monday morning, he never woke up." Rubina noted that she and her family were exhausted and were under a lot of emotional stress as they moved in and out of the hospital, nursing home, and palliative care unit.

Rubina feels that she was shortchanged on two accounts. First, she often wonders if her husband would still be alive if he had received the appropriate care when he first went to the hospital instead of "being sent home repeatedly from the hospital … every time we went, the doctors said he was alright." One cannot know whether race was a factor in this negligence; the literature suggests that difference comes into play, if not overtly then in subtle ways. The Canadian health care system is Eurocentric; its inclusion of racialized minorities is not an integral part of the system, but rather a form of patch-up work. Rubina carries the wound of not knowing whether the system was responsible for Navroz's death. This is the wound that will not heal. Second, she also felt wounded that the system did not provide adequate care for her husband. "It is us, the family, who had to take up complete responsibility for everything, not just emotional care."

Navroz's stay in the hospital, in the nursing home, and in the palliative unit only amounted to occupying physical space. Rubina takes solace in the fact that her family's care work revealed an ethics of care that the landscape of social palliation could include. Her inclusion of faith, spontaneous healing (Delya's daughter), and the holistic care provided by the family was healing for her husband, and this made it possible for him not to fall out of the world. Here, precarity was rendered into a resource.

Rubina shared her story because she wanted others to learn from her experiences. During our last meeting together, she informed me that she would be happy to talk to anyone to let them know more about how the system failed her. More important, she wished everyone to imbibe the quality of compassion, as her young grandson had done.

Through memory work five years after Navroz's death, Rubina reconfigures the meaning of a family-focused model of care. As for the health care system, Navroz fell between the cracks. It was his family who held his hand, to use the palliative care metaphor, to ensure that his dignity was maintained. Rubina's remembering of Navroz's life suggests an expanded model of care, one where medical diagnoses and faith are intertwined – elements for social palliation.

In her narrative, Rubina foregrounds a critical issue that might remain unnoticed were it not for the anthropological insight of the intertwined relationship between illness and socio-political conditions. In other words, it is not just the individual body but the body politic that matters. Livelihood is often regarded as fundamental to immigrants, forming the baseline for settlement. But this was not the case with Navroz. His wife explained that they had their own business and they were doing well financially. What Navroz missed was a network of social relationships, *anah dosht* (his peers). According to Michael Jackson (2006), the absence of networks can reduce a person to "mere objectivity, for this implies that he or she no longer exists in any active social relationship to others, but solely in the passive relationship to himself or herself, on the margins of the public realm" (45). We may ask, How did a situation come about that put Navroz in a position where he almost fell out of the world? As noted earlier, the primary reason is attributed to the fact Navroz found himself torn between two worlds: one (Kenya) that validated his status as a person, and another (Canada) that excluded him structurally to the extent that he did not acquire a sense of belonging, that is, a sense of being-in-the-world.

Rubina's narrative raises the larger question of what it means to be responsive to the ways in which the system hurts people. The events that led to Navroz's death are not concerns to be dismissed lightly: he fell between the cracks of the health care system; he did not receive timely treatment for a condition that proved to be fatal; his family was left to exclusively care for him; and his personhood was diminished. These concerns matter, and our attention to them allows us to see what we need to do to acquire a sense of belonging to the world – being-in-the-world. The latter aspect can be realized relationally and even intergenerationally, as in the case of Navroz's grandson. It is important to recognize other people's experiences as our own on the plane of vulnerability, as Butler (2012) has argued. This component forms part of the landscape of social palliation.

Shabina: Making a Case for Social Palliation

Shabina is among the few participants I met through an advertisement in an Iranian newspaper. She informed me that for her, as for many of her compatriots, the Iranian newspaper was an important source for keeping in touch with the world she had left behind. It was also an avenue through which this world was partially reconstituted by her being an "Iranian" in Canada. She felt that she did not belong to either of these worlds because her life revolved around her son, which was the reason she contacted me.

> I do not think that my son will receive the services that he is entitled to as a person with a disability. There is no one to advocate for him. After I pass away, I want my son to be comfortable and have quality of life.

It was on this note that Shabina told her story, explaining that she wanted to make a case for social palliation. Shabina stated at the outset that at the age of seventy-six, she is taking care of her forty-five-year-old son Navid. It is not normal for an aging mother to take care of an adult son; it should be the other way around. Highlighting the oddity of the situation, she creates a space for conversation with "whoever will listen."

Seated on a sofa along with Navid, Shabina enacted a critical event that happened many years ago in Iran. Using her hands, she explained how Navid fell from the bed when he was a baby. He did not cry but developed severe migraines that he has experienced all his life since then. He had a CT scan in Iran as well as in Canada. With the IQ of a fifteen-year-old, his condition has been diagnosed as incurable. Through her hands and tone of voice, Shabina stated that Navid is lovable, polite, and very giving. Through this performative gesture, she brings home an aspect often overlooked in the diagnosis of an incurable condition: she affirms his personhood. She feels sad that "he has missed out on all the joys of life; success from schooling, a satisfying job, marriage, and children." Putting her hand on his head, she continued, "If he has a migraine on a particular day, he will not be able to leave his room. He remains in the dark until the pain becomes less. When he is in pain, he gets frustrated." Shabina is a widow and has two other children in addition to Navid. The burden of care has been difficult on the family. "Both my son and daughter have dedicated their time and money to help him. Both are missing out from living their own lives. I am so tired mentally and physically."

"My son is undergoing palliative care"

Referring to our study on palliative care, Shabina said,

> I feel that my son is undergoing "palliative care." There is no cure for his disease. Instead, we give him medication and opportunities for social interaction to improve his quality of life. I believe care without hope or improvement of the illness should fall under palliative care. We wish to make his life as easy as we possibly can, giving him medicine and family support so he can live the way he pleases. I think this type of care should be patient-focused and should consistently take into consideration their wants and needs. To consent to what they want to do is giving them some control of their uncontrollable life.

Shabina advocates a broader baseline for palliative care, away from being a discrete unit. I have conceptualized the enactment of her story as memory work because of the way she relates it. She has made a choice not to "remember" her own life situation of becoming a widow or aging; neither does she talk about the lives of her other children except to state that the whole family is involved in taking care of Navid. This case of family-centred care raises a critical question: Should not the family-centred focus of palliative care be re-examined? Does this focus not echo the biomedical orientation of self-responsibility and self-care brought about by the restructuring of the health system? Importantly, Shabina's memory work – her construction of a life-course event linking Iran and

Canada through the body of her son – suggests that palliative care cannot be confined to the discrete space of the hospice or a medical setting.

The force of memory work comes to light through its capacity to relocate narratives of social suffering and anchor them to a politicized discourse. This shift requires a double vision, to use Das's (2003) term. Das notes, "Life and its forms are subjects of the political but then are remade at the level of the person" (294). Such a recognition makes the experience of suffering knowable. Shabina's memory work allows us to see how people find a voice to engage a listening audience, accomplishing two tasks. It makes us explore the point that people do not totally fall out of the world while at the same time it adds one more stroke to social palliation.

As I read through Shabina's transcript along with my field notes, I could hear her "voice" loud and clear. She calls for societal compassion and care. She gives the message

> I am old, and I am aging. I have taken care of my son for a lifetime. This situation cannot go on forever. One day, I am going to die. What will happen to my son? Who will take care of him? I cannot expect my daughter to take charge. She should also have a life.

It is at this moment that I realized that Shabina embodies familial wounds. She repeatedly stated that she and her daughter have "sacrificed" their lives for Navid. She does not know what will happen to him "after I am no longer in this world. Once I told my son, 'You should die with me. Nobody will provide for you emotionally,'" by which she means that no one will give him hugs, compassion, and holistic care. She stated that Navid's affectionate nature is not reciprocated. He greets everyone he sees, yet no one outside his family takes an interest in him. They return his greetings but do not engage him in a conversation. Shabina's battle is to make society validate his personhood.

Shabina was able to bring Navid to Canada only because she took on the responsibility of taking care of all his needs for a period of ten years. Although ten years of family sponsorship have passed, social services have not come forward to assist Navid, as Shabina had expected. Her disappointment is great. On one occasion when Navid was agitated, she observed, "You see, we do not have family here in Vancouver. If there was family, he would not be in this state. He needs people to talk to." As a sociable and compassionate person, Navid's loss upon migration to a new country is that of not having people to interact with.

Realizing the importance of people for Navid, Shabina sends him to produce stores near her house. "He can shop on his own," she states with pride. The underlying rationale is that these trips will enable him to engage into conversations with people. But she notes, "This does not happen. In Iran, it was different. People talk to you." Shabina has arranged for Navid to work for a private company. She pays them secretly so that Navid would be paid. "He feels good that he is earning," she notes with pride. To fill in the empty hours in the day, he "spends a lot of time on the computer, learning English and looking at different images."

"Citizenship Ethics"

Shabina bemoans the fact that her son has missed out on various joys of life. She feels that he should at least have the benefit of interacting with people. She tells me that Navid used to open the door for a female neighbour until she told him off with the words, "I have a husband," implying that Navid was making a pass at her.

Shabina is aware of Navid's medical condition, which she summarizes in the following way: "There is no cure for his disease. Instead we give him medication and opportunities for social interaction to improve his quality of life." Her tone of voice carries weight; the second part of the sentence is stated loudly and emphatically. This is the aspect that Shabina prioritizes. Opportunities for social interaction require a "citizenship ethic," to use Muehlebach's (2012) term, which must be worked for and nurtured. Shabina provides glimpses of this ethic based on her understanding of life. Consider the following three examples.

> I was watching the news and there was a segment showing how daycare centres were sending the children to visit nearby hospitals. They had taken twenty children to a hospital to visit elderly residents. They let the children spend the morning there. It was such a beautiful sight to see as the children, without hesitation, hugged the residents and drew pictures for them. Right away, you could see the joy and the sense of happiness exude from the residents. It was almost a form of therapy. *Patients/residents need to feel loved and respected as much as other people.* (emphasis added)

Shabina equates generational interaction with sociality. The children hugging the residents (a term she used interchangeably with patients) was appealing to her. Hugs do not occur easily in formal settings. For her, the joy and the happiness that was so palpable brought to light the principle that "patients need to feel loved and respected as much as other people." This is what she desires for her son.

The second example of a citizenship ethic comes across through Shabina's highlighting of Iranian cultural expectations. She notes, "if someone is ill, we try to comfort that person by holding his or her hand, showing affection through hugs and embraces. These physical gestures go a long way to make someone feel comfortable and valued." She continued, "By stroking their arms, you are showing that they have your attention and affection." Note that she does not use the term "patient" but rather the phrase "if someone is ill." The elements of hugging and holding hands form part of the citizenship ethic that requires "citizens to create the collective good through empathetic acts," performed in the public sphere (Muelbach 2012, 17). It is in this context that Sabrina related the third example, that of the fall of an elderly female neighbour.

> I immediately rushed towards her and put her head on my lap and began to stroke her. After arranging for the ambulance, I continuously tried to assure her that things would be alright in the best English words I could think of while holding her hand and stroking her head.

This "simple act of kindness," as Shabina put it, has led to the creation of an enduring friendship despite language barriers.

Shabina makes a case for social palliation for her son on two registers. First, she wishes to broaden the parameters of palliative care outside and beyond the discrete space of a physical facility such as hospice, hospital, or home. For her, this extended form of care must include citizenship ethics: the acknowledgment of one's personhood as realized in a world of social relationships. She gives the message that this quality cannot be realized in a situation where there is a divide between Us and Them. Her narrative recognizes the vulnerability and fragility of life. Second, she conveys the message that if Navid does not receive the quality care that would allow him to be part of the world, that is being-in-the-world, he will fall out of it upon her death.

Mobina: Social Precarity

How does a daughter remember her parents who have passed away? What message would she want to impart to a researcher exploring the issue of life, dying, and death? These are the questions I asked myself when I visited Mobina at the apartment that she shares with her husband. Mobina had prepared a spread of South Asian snacks that she served with *chai*. Pointing to a plate of *ghadiyah* (fried snack made from graham flour), she said, "My mother made very good *ghadiyah*. I get them from the store now that she is no longer in this world. This is my way of remembering her."

Mobina spoke fondly of her parents. She remembered her mother as "the kindest, most loving mother and grandmother, and a dedicated wife whose life centred around her husband." Her father was an entrepreneur in a small town in Tanzania.

> He had a clothes shop. He was very interested in clothes. Good appearance was important to him. He dressed well and expected the same of his children. He bought a pink *sari* [long, flowing South Asian attire] for my mother to wear on festive occasions.

She observed that back home, her patents had many friends, Hindus and Ismailis. They celebrated the Hindu festival of Diwali (festival of lights) and shared sweets with them. In fact, she continued, all the faiths mingled in the town where her parents lived. They participated in a lot of festivals and their socializing was an everyday activity.

Mobina's father, Zulfikar, ensured that all five of his children received a good education. He encouraged them to move abroad to advance their careers. Mobina described her parents' lives upon migrating to Canada as "uneventful," by which she meant that there were no festivals or robust social activity as they had been accustomed to in Tanzania.

> But they got on with their lives and were very happy in each other's company. They engaged into some activities such as playing board games, watching T.V. programs, and they enjoyed listening to classical Indian music and reading. They cooked together and ate together. They attended funerals [Ismaili] after which they would go out for a meal.

Then her father suffered a major stroke. According to Mobina, the active and healthy lifestyle her parents had cultivated for over a decade came to an end. "This proud, well-dressed man was unable to dress on his own. He stopped talking and became very quiet." Further conversations with Mobina revealed that the children took very good care of him. They travelled to be with him and decided that their father would never go into a nursing home. She recounted that her mother, Rehmet, looked after her husband and believed that he would make a full recovery. "When he passed away, she went into shock. She never shed a tear and never grieved. She stopped cooking and doing household chores." To help her mother heal, Mobina encouraged her to cook, but she was unsuccessful.

Because mum and dad always planned and cooked their meals together. Left on her own, my mother was lost. She had no routine anymore. She would not talk and whereas she had always been a hard-working woman all her life, she stopped doing anything.

All her children visited her, but she did not respond. Her son took her to the United States, where he lived. That did not help. The family discovered that Rehmet had developed early signs of Alzheimer's soon after her husband passed away. She would ask for her husband repeatedly, "*tara bapa kyare awse*" (when will your father come back?), and "*jo to bapa awi gaya*" (go and see if dad has arrived).

Mobina and her husband moved into Rehmet's apartment to take care of her. This situation lasted for seven years. The family decided to hire an Ismaili woman as a companion for their mother, since Mobina was working. But Rehmet's condition deteriorated. Mobina and her husband would find her walking at night, and often falling. Mobina addressed this issue by sleeping on a mattress in her mother's room. But it was difficult to take care of her because of her weight. "When she fell down it was difficult to lift her." Mobina relayed that she became stressed and that her health began to suffer. It was at this point that the family decided to move Rehmet to a care home. After the move, the family continued to take good care of her. Mobina and her husband visited her every day. They also ensured that she had a roommate. This way, when the roommate received visitors, they would also talk to Rehmet. "They would greet her and asked after her."

The care home was not a happy place for Rehmet. Mobina explained, "even though the care staff had been instructed that Rehmet was a vegetarian, they continued to make mistakes, giving her meat. The nurse would overlook to give her a bath or change her diapers. They did not take her out for regular walks." It is the absence of care that should make us question how care-work can be reduced to sheer abandonment, compromising one's humanity. In *Vita: Life in a Zone of Social Abandonment*, Biehl (2005) puts it this way, "You will see what people do to people. What it means to be human these days" (2). His interlocutor, Catarina, expressed the point, "And all of us together, we form a society, a society of bodies" (9). My observations in two care homes revealed that aging people with dementia felt abandoned by society and its institutions. Not wanting to generalize, many times I noticed that demented people were left in the lounge to "watch" TV for hours; in some cases, meals were brought to them so that the staff would not have to take them to the dining room, which would give them a change of environment. In Rehmet's case, the sense of being abandoned (giving meat to a vegetarian, not giving baths, and confining her to a room) was noted by the whole family. Mobina felt that "we were left to cope in whatever way we could. When I went into the kitchen to complain about the meat diet, I was told, 'the dietitian who takes care of these things is sick,' or 'she made a mistake and it will not happen again.'" But it happened over and over again despite the fact that, in Mobina's words, "The family had put up signs in her room specifying that she was a strict vegetarian and under no circumstances was she to be given any meat dishes." Mobina relayed the following incident,

> I remember the day when I was visiting my mum. A staff member was feeding her soup. Mum would look at it and shake her head and refused to eat it. She could see there were pieces of meat in the soup. The staff member insisted that she drink the soup. I asked her, "Do you know why she is not eating?" The staff member said, "Your mum is not keen on eating anything." I then pointed out to her that the soup had pieces of meat in it.

Other than the important matter of diet, two points are of interest. Mobina refers to the caregiver as a staff member. In other words, she sees her as someone who is just doing her job – bed-and-body work carried out in a manner that could be considered as deficient in not respecting Rehmet's dietary needs. Second, although Rehmet is dismissed as an Alzheimer's patient, and therefore a non-being, she is still aware that she is being given undesirable food and hence refuses to eat. Through this act, she speaks for other people with similar diagnoses: "We are but human though we have a different way of being-in-the-world."

Rehmet's world came apart long before her placement in the care home; it came apart because her social space had shrunk so much after migration that she could only share it with one person: her husband. Her world collapsed when he passed away. By way of contrast, Mobina portrayed her life in her homeland.

When she got up in the morning, the first thing she did was say her prayers. She would go to the living room and say, "Du'a [prayers] noh waqt thi gayo che. Chalo bada ahi avo, apne du'a padiye" (It is time for prayers. All of you come here, let us say du'a). When she called, the whole family gathered together. We all sat on the floor and my mother would recite the prayer. After breakfast, she planned meals for the day. She cut all the vegetables while interacting with other female members of the family. Whenever visitors, neighbours or other relatives dropped in, she would serve them tea with Indian snacks. She loved people. She was always warm and welcoming.

Mobina noted that her parents adjusted to their new life, but a closer look reveals that Zulfikar's hold on life was a struggle, and that Rehmet lived a life in-between the space of being-in-the-world and falling out of it. They adjusted to their new life, but this adjustment depended on establishing a daily routine *around each other, not the outside world*. What remained hidden was the fragility of their lives, and this would come to light at different moments. Zulfikar experienced this fragility in the moment when his life took an unexpected turn: from being an active person, he became one who remained silent in the wake of losing his ability to take care of himself. For Rehmet, the fragility of life was exposed when the precarious (limited) world that she had reconstituted fell apart following Zulfikar's death. It is her family who held on to the rope of life, not allowing it to break completely.

When I engaged Mobina in a conversation of how we could remedy a situation where her mother was treated as a non-person in the facility, she gave the example of a Sikh care home in Surrey. She noted that in this place, "residents" are treated as persons. This situation is a result of a paradigm shift from doing one's job to that of performing *seva* (service). She noted that residents are happy there and they have a long wait list. In *Aging and the Indian Diaspora*, Lamb (2009) observes, "Old age homes are viewed as appreciated sites of *seva*, respectful services towards elders." It is through seva that caregivers acquire a sense of satisfaction beyond the level of "just doing their job." This reciprocal concept, satisfying elders and caregivers simultaneously, could form an important component of social palliation.

Mobina noted: "All of us [the family] were left to take care of my mother in whatever way we could." She takes pride in the fact that her family, including her husband and grandchildren, "visited my mother, brought foods that she liked, watched photos with her and tried to keep her engaged." They did not allow Rehmet, a warm and welcoming person in her homeland, to fall out of the world.

While Mobina talked fondly of the care that her mother received from her extended family, she did not take the view that in her old age, she could expect kin-based care. Her observations are telling.

One should plan for one's future. You should proactively pick your own future home starting with assisted living homes. Do not leave it to the children. Plan it with your friends and go in as a couple. That way you do not get a shock when you are forced to live in a care home. Home [family home] can be very lonely. *The children have work and have their responsibilities and you are left alone for long periods of time in the home. It is not easy for the children to take you out or to Jamat Khana regularly either.* (emphasis added)

This is an unfolding story with a legacy whose presence will remain. This is because Mobina and her cohort are confronted with a dilemma: not being able to live in their own homes as they age but not accepting living with their children, not wanting to be a burden on them. Yet, they are convinced that somehow they will survive through their faith (*iman*), which Mobina considers a source of strength, resilience, and courage. Her life encapsulates precarity, encompassing vulnerability but also resourcefulness, which can be built into the palliation landscape.[3]

Legacies: Living and Dying

"Speak a new language so that the world will be a *new* world"

– Jalaluddin Rumi

Speaking through the language of metaphors, images, calligraphic art, memories, and the sounds and rhythms of sacred traditions, the following illustrations embody an existential question: What is it like to be awakened to human existence? An in-depth and close reading reveals that life and death are woven together in the lives of individuals and communities in a context that is inter-generational. Death is then perceived as part of lived realities unfolding over the course of life. I invite readers to reflexively expand the boundaries of these illustrations to include their repertoire of wisdom and wealth on uncertainty of life and certainty of death in the wake of displacement along with our attempts to fulfill socio-cultural and spiritual aspirations.

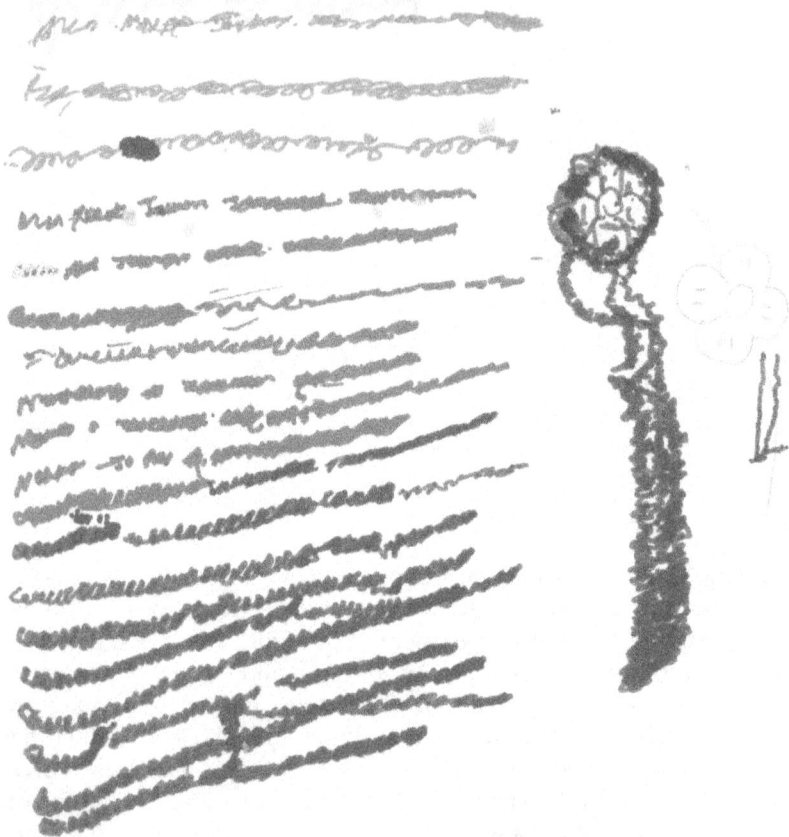

Figure 1 Last Breaths: Death in Life and Life in Death (Saker's drawing two weeks prior to her death)

When I am gone, release me, let me go:
I have so many things to see and do,
You must not tie yourself to me with tears,
Be thankful for our many years.

I gave you my love: you can only guess
How much you gave to me in happiness.
I thank you for the love you each have shown,
But now it's time I traveled on ... alone.

To grieve for me a while if grieve you must
Then let your grief be comforted by trust.
It's only for a time that we must part:
So bless the memories within your heart.

I won't be far away, for life goes on: so
If you need, call and I will come: though
You can't see me or touch me, I'll be near and if
You listen with your heart you will hear all
My love around you, soft and clear.

And then when you must come this way alone,
I'll greet you with a smile and say 'welcome home'.

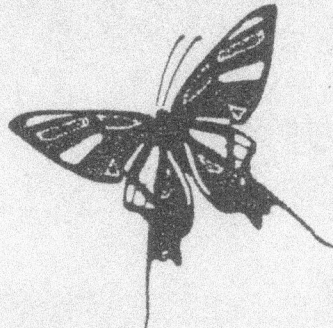

Figure 2 "To Those I Love": Last Words for My Husband

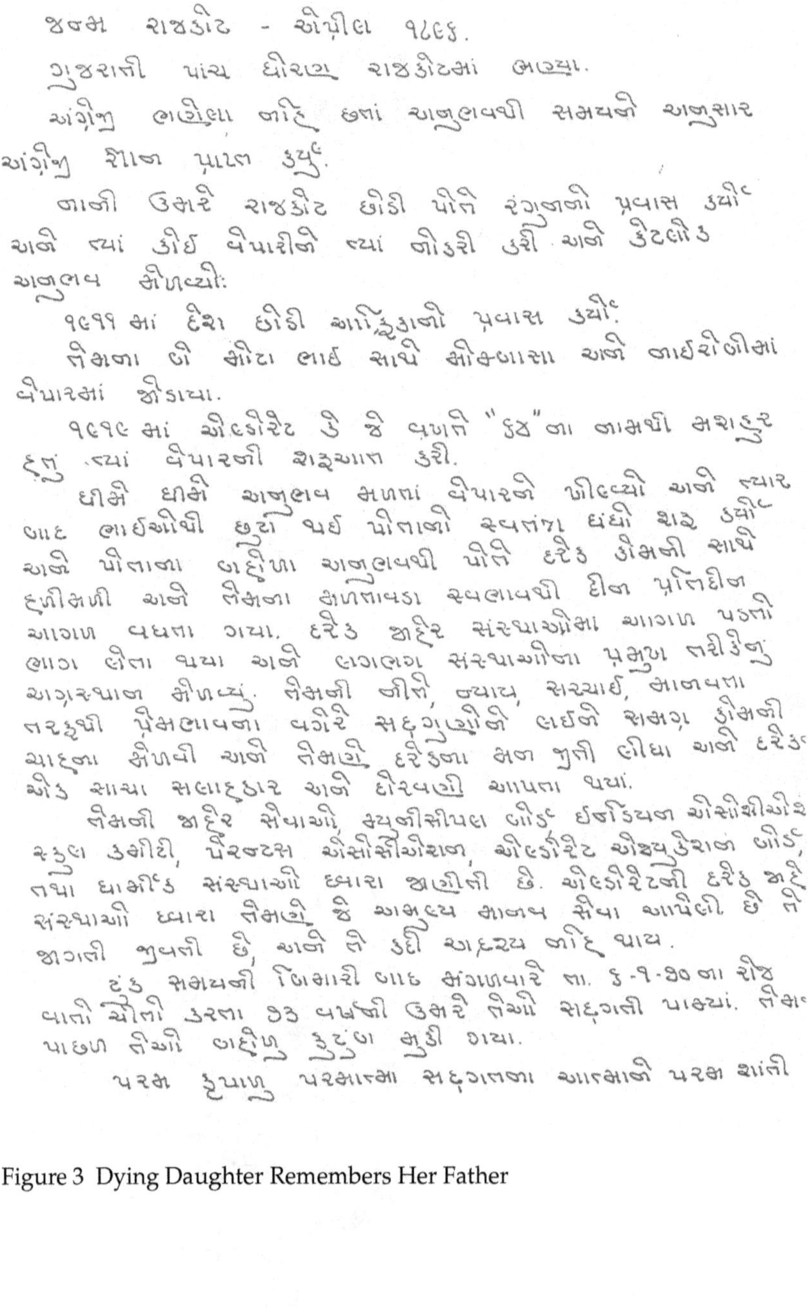

જન્મ રાજકોટ - એપ્રીલ ૧૮૬૬.

ગુજરાતી પાંચ ધોરણ રાજકોટમાં ભણ્યા.

અંગ્રેજી ભણેલા જાહે છતાં પાછલવયી સમયની આજ્ઞાસાર અંગ્રેજી રીજ પ્રાણ કર્યું.

જાવી ઉમરે રાજકોટ છોડી પોતે રંગુનનો પ્રવાસ કર્યો અને ત્યાં કોઈ વેપારીને ત્યાં નોકરી કરી અને કેટલોક આજ્ઞાબ મેળવ્યો.

૧૯૧૧ માં દેશ છોડી આફ્રીકાનો પ્રવાસ કર્યો.

તેમના બે સીતા ભાઈ સાથે સીક્ખાસા અને નાઈરોબીમાં વેપારમાં જોડાયા.

૧૯૧૯ માં ઓલડોરેટ કે જે વખતે "કટ"ના નામથી ઓશાહુર હતું ત્યાં વેપારની શરૂઆત કરી.

ધીમે ધીમે આજ્ઞાબ સાથનાં વેપારને ખીલવ્યો અને ત્યાર બાદ ભાઈઓથી છૂટા પઈ પોતાનો સ્વતંત્ર ધંધો શરૂ કર્યો અને પોતાના બાહુળા આજ્ઞાબવયી પોતે દરેક ઓમની સાથે હમીકામ અને તેમના આગળાવડા સ્વભાવયી દીન પ્રતિદીન આગળ વધતા ગયા. દરેક જાહેર સંસ્થાઓમાં આગળ પડતા ભાગ લેતા વયા અને લગભગ સંસ્થાઓના પ્રમુખ તરીકે આગ્રસ્થાન મેળવ્યું. તેમજી જીતી, ન્યાય, સચ્ચાઈ, આબાનના તરફથી પ્રેમભાવના વગેરે સદ્ગુણોને લીધે સઘળા ઓમની આહ્મા મેળવી અને તેમને દરેકના હ્મ જુગી લીધા અને દરેક એક સાચા સલાહ્દાર અને દોરવણી આપતા વયા.

તેમની જાહેર સેવાની સ્મૃતીસીપલ બોર્ડ ઈર્જીડીયલ ઓસીસીઓસ રકુલ ઉકીડી, પેરવટસ ઓસીસીઓસેશ, ઓલડોરેટ ઓય્ચભેરાજ બોર્ડ, તથા ધાર્મીક સંસ્થાઓ દ્વારા જાણીતી છે. ઓલડોરેટની દરેક જાહે સંસ્થામાં દ્વારા તેમને જે આબ્હ્ય આબન્ય સેવા આપેલી છે તે જાગતી જુવતી છે, અને તે કદી આદર્ય નાહે થાય.

ટૂક સમયની બિમારી બાદ સંગાળવારે તા. ૬-૧-૭૦ ના રોજ વાતી એોની ઉરતા ૭૩ વર્ષની ઉમરે તેઓ સદ્ગતી પામ્યા. તેમ પાછળ તેઓ બાહ્યોળ કુટુંબ મુકી ગયા.

પરમ કૃપાળુ પરમાત્મા સદ્ગતના આત્માને પરમ શાંતી

Figure 3 Dying Daughter Remembers Her Father

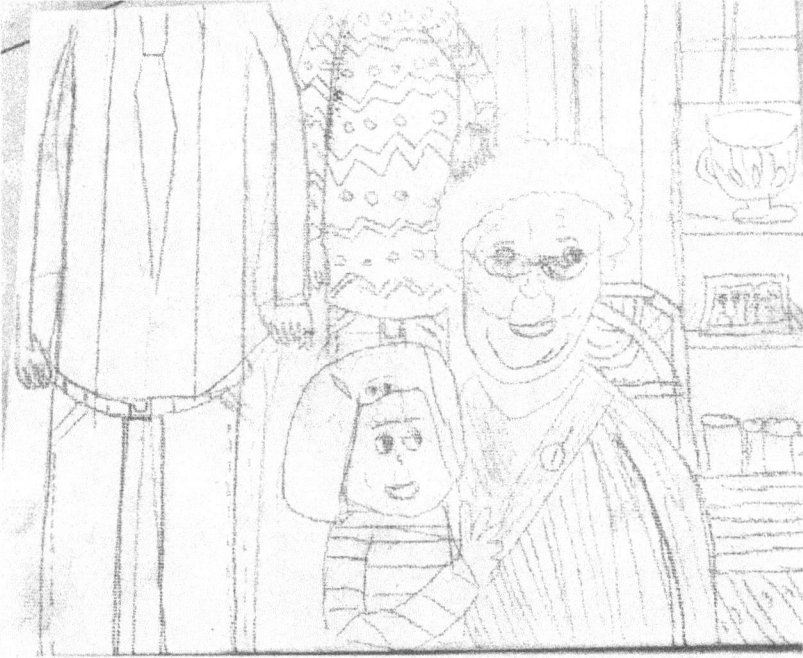

"Those who left are not lost, for before she left she planted a seed of memory and watched as it grew of all the past love she felt for you, so take heed. Those who wander away are not lost for they have a home in your heart and nothing that ever happens can rip that home apart".

******

"The hope that glowed fell in the black, for the loved one is gone and their presence you lack; a journey up to the star but now you are alone and your loved one is far, you've cried and begged and now you groan, but when you look up at the star, you are not alone".

Figure 4   Ten-Year-Old Zoe Pays Tribute to Her Nanima (Grandmother)

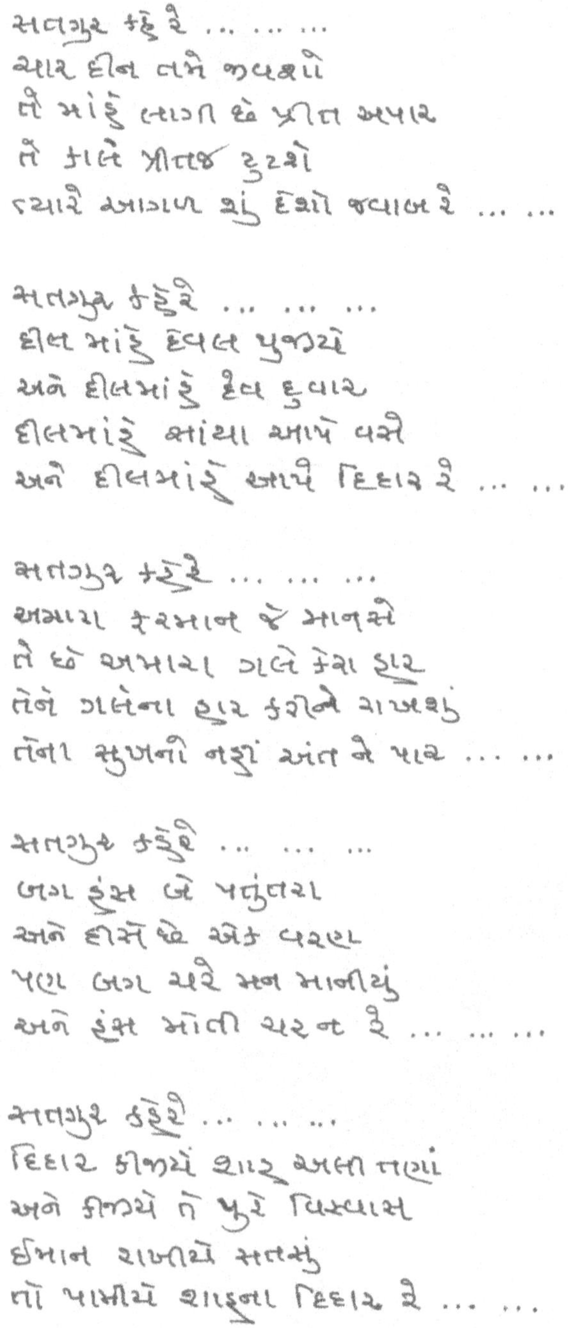

સતગુર કહે રે ... ...
આર દીન તમે જવશો
તે માંહે લાગી છે પ્રીત અપાર
તો મારે પ્રીતજ દૂરશે
ત્યારે આગળ શું દેશો જવાબ રે ... ...

સતગુર કહે રે ... ...
દીલ માંહે દેવલ પુજવું
અને દીલમાંહે દેવ દુવાર
દીલમાંહે સાંયા આપે વસે
અને દીલમાંહે આપે દિદાર રે ... ...

સતગુર કહે ... ...
અમારા ફરમાન જે માનસે
તે છે અમારા ગલે ફેરા હાર
તેને ગળેના હાર કરીને રાખશું
તેના સુખની નહીં અંત ને પાર ... ...

સતગુર કહે ... ...
જગ હંસ બે પતુંરા
અને દીસે છે એક વરણ
પણ જગ ચરે મન માનીયું
અને હંસ મોતી ચરન રે ... ...

સતગુર કહે રે ... ...
દિદાર કીજયે શાહ અલ્લા તણાં
અને કીજયે તો પુરે વિસ્વાસ
ઈમાન રાખીયે સતસું
તો પામીયે શાહના દિદાર રે ... ...

Figure 5 Sacred Traditions: Verses from Ginans (Scripted by Sadru)

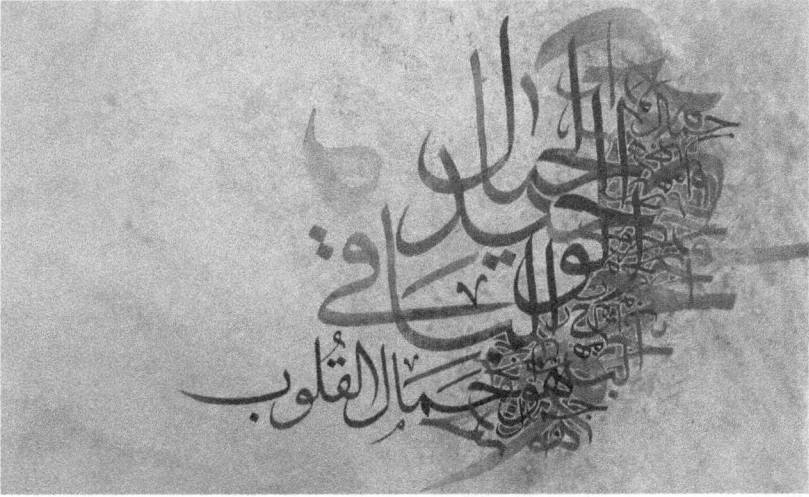

Figure 6   Sacred Traditions: Calligraphic Representations of Verses from Jalaludin Rumi (*The only remaining beauty is the beauty of hearts*). By Khaled Al-Saa'i.

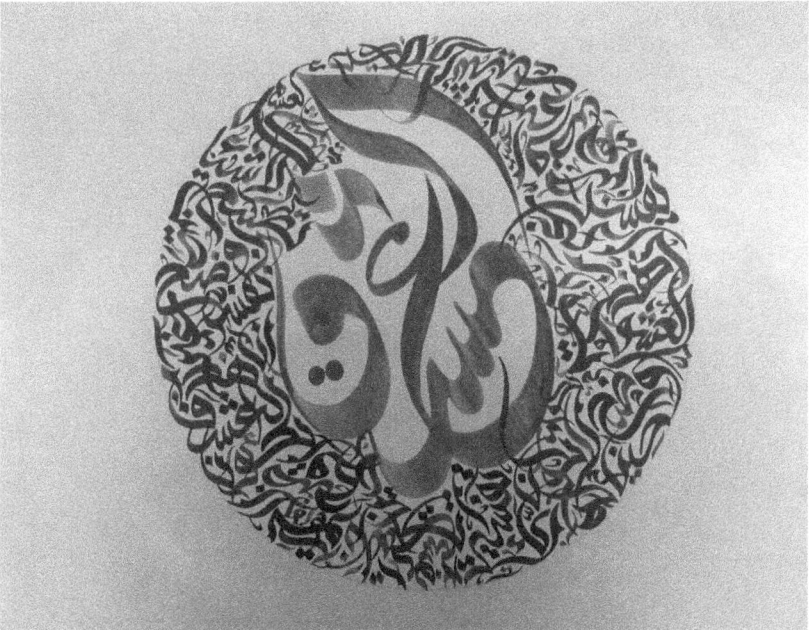

Figure 7   Sacred Traditions: Calligraphic Representations of Verses from Jalaludin Rumi (*Everything in this universe gets clear when explained, but this love is clear with no explanation*). By Khaled Al-Saa'i.

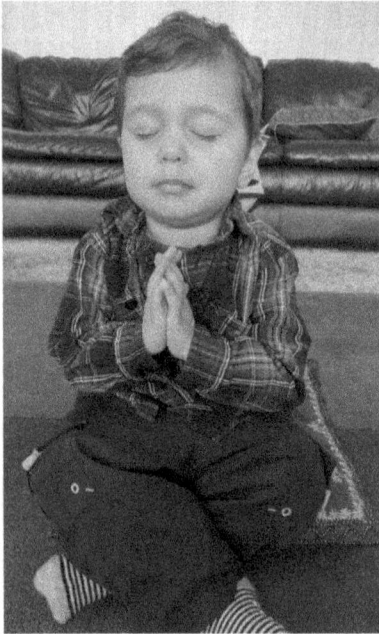

Figure 8 Intergenerational Transmission of Sacred Traditions: Isaan.

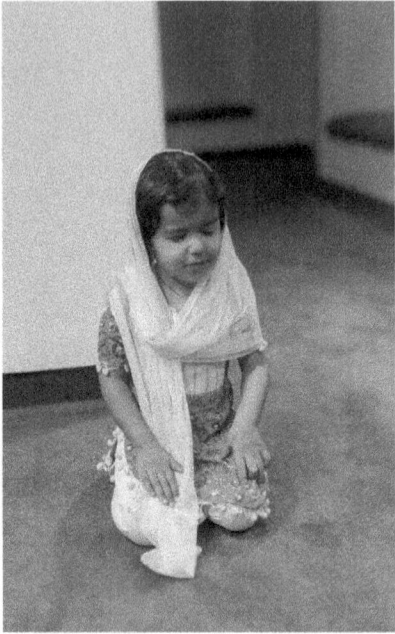

Figure 9 Intergenerational Transmission of Sacred Traditions: Zoey.

PART 2

4 Re-making a Home in the Diaspora[1]

We may ask: What is the connection between re-making a home and life and death? By now we may have figured out that there is a deep connection between the two for the simple reason that death is not a discrete phenomenon. It is enmeshed in life. What is fascinating about death is that it lends itself to different forms of articulation, the contours of which can be embedded in social palliation. Both life and death can be expressed in ritual, poetry and art, and ordinary everyday conversations, where talk on the passing away of a relative or a close friend is not uncommon. The anchor of this phenomenon is the home, which may be material, imagined, and/or narrativized. Re-making a home, informed by the foundation narrative of life and death, is of special relevance to diasporic people for whom this endeavour assumes special significance; having "lost" a home, their efforts to reconfigure another one are structurally constrained, as was the case with my study participants.

Two questions were uppermost in the minds of the participants as they sought to re-make a home: first, what kind of life would it enable them to lead and how would this life resonate with death? Second, how would they transmit their experiential understanding of life and death to the younger generation, who had been brought up in a different milieu? The participants understood that life and death does not constitute a subject that can merely be talked about. During our conversations, they noted that this fundamental matter unfolds gradually and over time; what was needed was a world of social relationships where issues of life and death could be learned through concrete realities, relayed within the space of a home and its interconnection to the wider world. I have thus organized this chapter, and the next one, as follows. Following an overview of the literature on the diaspora and re-making a home, I present vignettes from my journal entries, laying the groundwork for the storied lives of women keen to talk about this issue with vigour. Given their social positionality in the diaspora, they felt the need to articulate their life experiences. The women gave me to understand that it is only through an appreciation of living and dying in a "foreign" place that their lives would be acknowledged in terms of who they were in their home countries (social status) and what has become of them in Canada (loss of social status attributed to racialization entangled with neoliberalism and aging). I argue that re-making a home ultimately relates to life and death as an integral unit. Understanding this requires that home be connected to a world of social relationships, a refrain put forward by the study participants. I ask the question, What are the implications for living and dying if such a connection is ruptured?

Overview: Diasporic Home

Diaspora scholars have highlighted the multiple meanings that home has assumed since its original conceptualization as forced displacement from a homeland (Agnew 2005; Castillo 2012; Hua 2005; Ray 2004; Pasura 2013). In this age of global migration, the term diaspora evokes transborder identities (Joseph 2013), reconfiguration of gender and kinship (López 2012), reconstruction of home and intimate relations (Boehm 2012), formation of hybrid identities (Duruz 2005), and the politics of food (Mankekar 2002). "Understanding diasporic formations can help us comprehend the relocation and community-making of those people who were previously oppressed and colonized, as well as those who are forced to – or choose to – stay put back home" (Hua 2005, 191). Despite its potential to enrich lives through acquiring what I call border-knowledge from two or more countries, diasporas capture a paradox as they "exist in tension with the norms of nation-states and with nativist identify formations" (192). Joseph (2013) puts it this way, "Knowledge, skills and cultural resources of immigrants that are underutilized in the receiving nations have detrimental social and economic effects on immigrants' communities and the nation-state" (35). Faced with prejudice and hostility from the host society, diasporic subjects/migrants reconfigure their lives under constraints and structural limitations, such as securing a livelihood or negotiating the health system (Pasura 2013).

In short, immigrants experience tensions and contradictions arising from socio-economic exclusions in Canada, notwithstanding the less than amicable environment in their homelands. The latter may be a function of economic displacement, political situation, religious persecution, and/or war and violence. Drawing upon cultural and social resources from transnational/borderland spaces, immigrants actively engage in re-making a home; this process "can help one to understand the social world resulting from displacement, flight, exile, and forced migration" (Hua 2005, 196). Study participants experienced life in the diaspora more in the form of ruptures. My choice of the stories relayed by Canadian-Iranian and Canadian Ismaili-Muslim study participants, aged forty-five and over, is informed by their ruptured experiences of re-making a home. It was within this space that they sought to convey their understanding of life and death, grounded in their experiences of everyday life and its fragility, as noted in the vignettes below.

Diasporic Ruptures

Vignette 1: Food

> There was a time when I had a place on a table full of people and a presence as part of other food dishes, especially my companion, the curry. It gave me a good feeling that I satisfied so many people. I remember being kneaded into a dough and divided into small portions by a nurturing hand. I was then rolled into round shapes and roasted on a special pan called *tawdhi* (special pan). The pan was reserved for me only. Now that I have crossed the border into another country, my use is limited to once or twice in a week. My pan sits alone in the corner of a kitchen shelf. It is no longer included in the everyday activities that take place in the kitchen. I feel good when occasionally my nurturer uses me to make twenty *rotlis* that are distributed to her children. They take me to their homes, but they do not consume me right away when I am fresh and desirable. They put me in the freezer, an unpleasant experience that I never had before. When they are ready to include me in their meal, they put me in a microwave. Freezing cold to very hot in a matter of minutes. I leave it to your imagination as to what this process is like given that it occurs in minutes. Sometimes I find myself in the microwave twice when the children are late for a meal owing to the busyness of their lives. When the parents eat alone, I feel their loneliness. They do not enjoy me as much when the children are not present. I am no longer whole as I once was. I can express myself in language only because of my experience of rupture. I no longer exist in a house full of people who would relish me. My experience of being frozen (alone and isolated) enables me to put into words my feelings of being cut off from the world I once knew intimately.

As I tried to understand the implication of this shift from a popular item to that of a rare one, two points came to mind. First, the Gujarati term *rotlis* connotes abundance as these are made in batches and rarely as one piece. Rotlis are consumed and prepared for more than one person. Being plural connotes its consumption in a world of social relationships of kith and kin. Second, a different situation prevails in the Canadian diaspora with its orientation towards nuclear family units. If rotlis were to "speak," they would bemoan the loss of relationships, the context that sustains them.[2]

Vignette 2: Flowers

Consider a vase of flowers placed on a kitchen table, a scene I often came across during my interviews with women. I often found flowers to be fading at various stages in their lives. Some were relatively fresh while others were drooping and yet others were shedding their petals. Surrounding the flowers were evergreens. Each flower has its own story, the foundation of which would be the soil in which it grew, the amount of sunshine and water it received along with tender care or its lack, and the way in which it was plucked. The flowers speak to us about life and death. At one time, they were fresh and desirable. Now as they are fading, they are looked upon with different eyes with the view that they will be disposed of soon. We need to pause and pay attention to their silent message. Each flower enhances the colours, the shapes, and the textures of the others telling a collective story of how singular lives relate to others without losing their distinguishing characteristics. Each flower stands out in relation to the other. By itself, it would appear to be dead. An important aspect is that of the green leaves being there for the fading flowers to support them. This vignette stands by itself for the reader to glean its message about sociality and interconnectivity.

The above reading made me realize that although we cannot capture the full range of human experiences, some aspects can be made comprehensible. As I continued with my field research, I realized that vignettes and singular stories effect a shift from an "I" to a "We." The "We" embodies intergenerational relationships and the network of relationships integral to what makes us human. It is the "We" aspect that the protagonists of the stories found wanting. Nevertheless, they directed their efforts to re-make a home and draw out its significance for life and death, as part of living, a subject matter that is not articulated discursively but is not far from the surface. Lambek (2016) observes, "Most people do know something about death from the personal experience of losing friends and family or witnessing death in road accidents, wars, or hospitals, and possibly also from personal intuition" (629).

It is within the space of a diasporic home that the subject matter of death is broached in the context of undertones, such as, "One day we are going to die"; "We are not going to take anything with us. We came into this world with empty hands and we will go with empty hands," said Maryam, when I expressed my condolences on the death (*marg*) of her sister in Iran. Home is the place where the death of a family member is commemorated. On this occasion, kin and peers get together for prayers and ceremonies. The "conversion" of a home into a place of mourning comes into relief through the medium of food. No cooking takes place until the burial has occurred. Food, forming part of the mourning ritual, is brought into the home by relatives for consumption by kith and kin. Also, prayers for the soul of the deceased are performed within the space of the home. In the case of Ismailis, home is connected to the Jamat Khana; for the Iranians, home is connected to a dense network of kin ties. This does not mean that the house of prayer or kin ties are absent for both communities. I make my observation by way of emphasis. The period of mourning varies from one week to forty days; the latter may be condensed given the busyness of life, as noted above.

The conversion of the diasporic home into a space for mourning reveals a stark reality. Following the death of a family member, one's home is by and large filled with people, including relatives who may have travelled from other parts of the world to pay their respects. Once the ceremonies are over, one's home, in the words of a participant, "becomes empty." A grieving widow informed me that in the presence of people, she did not feel the loss of her husband until everyone had left. *"Hawe mane bohu sunu sunu lageh che"* (now I feel very very alone).

The above scenario, common to both communities, illustrates that dilemmas and contradictions constitute the process of re-making a home in the diaspora, a perspective advanced by scholars such as Gilmartin and Migge (2015), Long (2013), Warin and Dennis (2008), and Tsolidis (2011). Citing the example of two British Palestinian women, Ilfat and Wadad, respectively, Long (2013) observed that neither of them felt at home until they had created social and affective spaces – spaces that enabled them to have a sense of belonging, not excluding rootlessness, that exceeded territorial boundaries. Using the term "politics of diasporic dwelling," Long observes, "Domestic space is a dialectic of inside and outside, of house and the universe, of intimacy and the world in the *fundamental interconnectedness of people and places through imagination*" (335, emphasis added).

The interconnectedness of places and people are what my research participants sought in their search to re-make a home. A primary issue that study participants encountered when they migrated was the norm of the nuclear family unit, integral to neoliberal capitalism, with its emphasis on individualization. The on-the-ground realization of this norm was twofold. At one level, it entrenched the idea, in the words of fifty-two-year-old Farida, that "homes in Canada are built for mother, father and their children. If our parents live with us, it is considered as something special, not part of how things should be." This is indeed the case because older people living with their children feel that they are a burden. "We never used to have this kind of feeling back at home. Here is the photo of my house in Dar es Salaam (Tanzania). Does this kind of a house give the message that it is only meant for parents and their children?" noted eighty-two-year-old Fatma during our conversation on the meaning of home. It is important to note that nuclear family units translate into restricted and diminished social spaces. Fifty-eight-year-old Farah noted, "If there are more people in the home, there is more activity as people come in and go out. This is how it was in my country. You always see people in and out. Here, this is not the case. When I look at my neighbours' homes, I get the sense that no-one lives there. There are hardly any activities outside these homes." It is in the context of everyday and homely interactions and activities that one acquires an understanding of what it is like to live and what it is like to die.

Deploying the term "gated communities," Low (2001, 2011) argues that such communities promote new forms of exclusion in residential settings. As the elite in urban and suburban areas retreat into enclaves, walls and gates create barriers to social interactions and forming social networks. Retreating into one's own domestic space, she continues, invariably leads to an intolerance of diverse groups demarcated along the lines of race, gender, age, religion, and class. This milieu informed study participants' restorative but also ruptured work of re-making a home in the diaspora.

The first generation of Canadian-Iranians and Canadian Ismaili-Muslims, by and large, had lived in joint families, though not without conflict. These families embodied a world of social relationships where knowledge of what it means to live and what it means to die was acquired in a way that was intimate and transmitted over a period of time. This understanding is not fostered fully within nuclear family units because their social space is so diminished. "How did women go about sustaining the foundation story of life and death in the process of re-making a home in the diaspora?" is the question I asked in my interviews and conversations with participants from both the communities. In other words, how is a home reconstituted (even if it is ruptured) with the intent of giving meaning to life and death? Participants' responses

were substantiated through stories and memory work: Homa and Firouzeh from the Canadian-Iranian community, and Tamiza, Zarina, and
Sabrina (continued in chapter 5) from the Canadian Ismaili-Muslim
community.[3] My choice of these narratives is based on the enthusiasm
of the participants to share their stories, exemplified by Firouzeh as:
"This is our opportunity to tell it all. No one has shown interest in our
lives." These singular narratives encapsulate a collective scenario.

Homa: "I have a story to tell"

These are the words that Homa uttered soon after I had gone through
the ethics protocol form for Simon Fraser University. I was struck as to
how keen she was to share her story within the space of her "home."
She considered stories a medium for exploring the ultimate issues of
life: its meaning and valuation, the process of aging, and who would
care for her when she approached the end of her life. Gesturing with her
hands, Homa relayed the following account.

> I have a story to tell. My story is about not having a proper home. Soon
> after I came to Canada, we discovered that my husband, who is a pedia-
> trician, will not have work in Canada. This was difficult for us to hear.
> The immigrant officer had informed us that we would have no problems
> in securing work. I am a nurse. My husband was told that he could go
> back to school to get "Canadian" qualifications. This was impossible. We
> had two children attending primary school. We came to Canada for their
> education. He went back to Iran to earn a living. I stayed behind to raise
> the children. As my children grew older, I started looking for work. They
> [employment office] asked me to do volunteer work. This way they said,
> "I would get 'Canadian qualifications' [*emotional tone; gesturing with the
> hands to emphasize her point but also to point out the unfairness of a situation
> where she could not find work despite her qualifications and fluency in English*].
> I was going crazy staying at home. I decided to do volunteer work but
> even this was hard. Eventually, I worked as a volunteer for English as a
> Second Language (ESL) Program, set up for Iranians. My job was to do
> translation back and forth between Farsi and English. Seeing that I was
> good, they [the program officer] hired me part-time. I do not think it was
> part-time work. The Iranian women would phone me at home and talk
> to me soon after ESL classes were over. They had so many issues. This
> required finding out what services they could access. Sometimes they just
> wanted to talk about their problems. I was working full time without pay.
> It was all right. At least I was doing service work, the reason I took up the
> nursing profession.

My husband would come over whenever he got vacation time. I also visited him with the children. We moved back and forth between Canada and Iran. Once it was Nurooz [Iranian New Year, 22 March]. My husband could not come. The children were so disappointed. *We did not celebrate Nurooz, the most important occasion for us* [emphasis in the original]. When the children became older, we decided to send them to the United States for further education. I stayed in the apartment that we had bought in Vancouver. This way the children could visit us, and their father could visit us at the same time. It was important for our family to meet two or three times a year. Now my children are married and settled in the United States. One is married to a white American and the second one is married to an Iranian girl. I cannot consider Vancouver to be my home. I have spent many empty hours in the apartment with no family members around. I had Iranian friends but they were also my "clients." We will keep the apartment for family get together[s]. We rarely go to the United States to visit our children. They come to Vancouver. I am aging. Once I reach old age and need care, I will go back to Iran. What I have there is family and friends though many of them have left the country like we did. My home in my old age will be Iran. *This is where I wish to die* [emphasis in the original].

When I asked Homa to state the meaning of home, she explained, "In Iran, our house was not so big, but it appeared big because we had so many visitors. In Canada, our apartment appears to be spacious as it was just me and my children. Iran was more like home. Presently our Canadian apartment is "empty" because the children are gone. In Iran, some of the relatives and many of our friends have migrated; but still there are people you can interact with daily. For me then home is here and there." She drew a picture of two homes, one with people (Iran) and another one (Canada) that was relatively empty.

In the intimate space of the home

Homa, like many of the women I had come to know well, invited me to her residence. When I entered, she had two large pots on the stove along with plastic Tupperware. Upon inquiring why she was making so much food, she said, "I am going to Iran to see my husband. The children will be here. I will freeze the food for them." Pointing to the extra Tupperware placed on the opposite counter, she informed me that she was going to take these to Iran. "Before I return, I will cook food for my husband and freeze it for him to eat while I am away." Homa takes plastic Tupperware to Iran because "the Canadian-made is sturdy for freezing food. I bring spices from Iran. When I bring packages of spices, my children ask me the names; they like to smell them. Have you used saffron that comes from Iran? It is the best in the world. The aroma it gives is soothing." More than gendered work, Homa's cooking constitutes cultural labour. Cultural labour goes beyond the act of feeding and nourishing. It is through cultural labour that Homa re-makes a home with a focus on life and living, underpinned by dying and death.

Her starting point is recognizing the dilemmas her children are faced with as to the question "Where is home?" Realizing that language is key to understanding home and its connection to life and its unfolding on the plane of death, she and her husband talk to the children in Farsi. During my conversation with her after she completed an ESL class, she observed, "Here I am encouraging Iranian women to speak English. When I go home, I encourage my children to speak Farsi. More and more, they are using English." Homa is confronted with a contradiction that is structural. Her assigned task is to ensure that the Iranian women she works with learn English so that they can "integrate" into Canadian society. However, promoted by the state and its institutions, integration amounts to downplaying the value system and traditions of racialized minorities in the public sphere (for example: Agnew 1997; Bannerji 1995; Dossa 2004).

On the home front, Homa notes that her children have internalized the hegemonic norm of English being valued more than heritage languages. She is aware of the peer pressure school exercises. She tells me that even if the parents talk to the children in Farsi, the children talk to each other in English. It is a subtle shift that she noticed over time. She takes consolation in the fact that food is one area that is not subject to substitution and translation. Her children ask her to make dishes such as *tahdig* (crunchy fried rice), *bademjan* (eggplant in tomato stew), *kebab* (made from ground lamb and other meats), *nan* (flat bread) and *shabji* (herbs and vegetables). "They never use English names. It would sound funny," she commented while sharing a kebab with me.

Scholars on food have informed us that food embodies culture, history, and memories (Kadar 2005; Lind and Barham 2004; Mankekar 2002; Smith and Jehlička 2007).

Preparing and consuming food has emotional, symbolic, and social significance. For immigrants, food contains a world of their imagining of what life had been like and what it is becoming. Like people, food crosses borders, and in doing so carries elements from the past while accommodating others from the present. But the process is not smooth, as immigrant families negotiate which aspects of foodways to maintain and which ones to let go as they go about re-making a home in the wake of structural constraints. This does not rule out the process of adaptation (Dyck and Dossa 2007).

Food preparation has not been easy for Homa. While she takes pride in feeding her family even when she is not around (frozen food), she is keenly aware that she (not her husband) had to give up her profession, for which she worked very hard. On one occasion, as we were having coffee, an older Iranian woman walked in who knew Homa. She came to our table and informed her that her daughter had just graduated as a nurse. While Homa congratulated (*mobarak*) her, I could feel her pain. When I asked her later as to why she did not seem to be happy, she said, "Umm I wish I had gone back to school here [in Canada], then I would also be practicing my profession." After some time, she added, "But how could I have. My children were small [*hand gesture*]. I could not leave them alone especially when my husband was not here." I want to acknowledge the social weight that Homa carried on her shoulders, placed on her because of an accreditation barrier that immigrants (read racialized minorities) encounter when they migrate to Canada. Life would have been very different for Homa and her family if the couple's professions had been recognized in Canada; they had more than fifteen years of experience in their home country.

Homa's cooking was not free of what I have referred to as diasporic ruptures. Once, as we were going through her photo album, she showed me a picture of a well-laid table, with cutlery and plates nicely arranged and a couple of Iranian dishes placed at the centre. She noted, "This is how we used to have our meals. Table laid and variety of dishes that we enjoyed as a family. We all had stories to tell each other. My husband and I talked about our work and the children brought news from school. Here, it is not the same. I no longer lay the table. What is the use? My husband is in Iran, the children are in school and they have after-school activities. Sometimes I eat alone and sometimes I wait for them. Many times, the food is warmed up in the microwave." Homa feels that other than service work (the ESL program), cooking gives her satisfaction but not as much as day-to-day work. She does not enjoy shopping, cooking, and cleaning on her own. She observed, "My children will remember me because I feed them not only when I am here but also when I am in Iran [frozen food]." Evoking aroma, taste, touch, and feel, food forms part of memory that is not easily erased. Memories may go under the surface but may be recalled in the context of everyday life and on festive occasions. Homa is convinced that her food-work will be appreciated and remembered by her children when she is no longer in this world. "Many times, when I see them or talk to them over the phone, they tell me how much they value the food I prepare for them, fresh or frozen."

It was only when I got to know Homa well that I broached the subject of end-of-life, as was the case with the other women. As noted earlier, I wanted to understand the relationship between this phase of life and re-making a home. Homa's response was telling: "You see, we have not been able to make a home in Canada. Home is where the family is. Except for the times when my husband visits, I have been alone with the children. When the children left for the United States for their education, I was all by myself except when I spent time in Iran with my husband, family, and friends. This was when my children were older. We have kept our apartment here. We are Canadian citizens. We need to keep our citizenship. If I fall sick or when I reach old age, I will go back to Iran. I think this is the country where I would like to die surrounded by people. I dread the idea of being alone in Canada even if my husband was here."

When I asked her if she would consider living with her married children, she said, "They love me, and they would take care of me. But you know if they were to take care of me, they will not respect (*ehteram*) me as much as they do now. I would be a burden on them. We cannot be a burden on them. Umm you know they have busy lives. In Iran, I would have more than one person taking care of me; my sisters and my aunts live there. The burden of one person doing care work would be spread." Homa is also concerned that if she lived with her children, they would not be able to serve her Iranian food. She would be too old to cook. Food, she informed me, was critical to her well-being, symbolically and socially. It was a connecting thread in her life as she had childhood memories of her mother's cooking, festive occasions when families got together, and everyday consumption when "no one ate alone as they do here. I do not want to eat burgers and pasta when I grow old. These are the foods you can eat by yourself," she noted.

I wrote in my diary, "Here is a couple who came to Vancouver to set up a home. Their efforts are filled with ambiguity. They have a physical home but not a social one. In other words, they are Canadian citizens without a home in the affective sense. They have not been able to secure substantive citizenship that would include a basic right: the right to work in one's area of expertise. Homa will eventually go back but not without interrogating the boundaries of the nation-state. She belongs to two splintered worlds: Iran, where she has access to the world of social relationships (diminished to some extent because of transmigration) and Canada, where, as a citizen, she is entitled to health and other services devoid of personal touch. Her home is split between these two countries. This split speaks to the anomaly of tightly knit boundaries of the nation-state." Homa observed, "Although my children are in the

United States, they understand the meaning of home as being a place for family to live and be together. They tell me that they will look after me when I grow old. But I do not agree to that. I do not want to be a burden." She "lives" in Vancouver to keep her family together. But this is not the place where she wishes to die. "Homing the city," to use Low's and Merry's term (2010) – the existence of a dense network of social relationships – would be the space to sustain the integrity of life and death, a pathway for social palliation.

Firouzeh: "Just because we have lost the use of our legs, this does not mean that we do not have brains"

If you were to meet Firouzeh, you would be struck by her resilience. She is adept at using her wheelchair; she moves around swiftly and gracefully. The wheelchair became part of her being following an accident when she was in her teens. At the time, she lived in a village in Iran. Sensing that she would be a burden on her family, she opted to go to Tehran (city), where she found work in a sewing factory. It was here that she met her husband, Hossein, also a wheelchair user. Firouzeh took pride in the fact that their wedding picture appeared in the newspaper as this was the first time that there was a marriage of "two people in wheelchairs." The couple raised four children. Of interest is Firouzeh's account of how she accomplished this task. First and most important, it was her conviction that, "just because we have lost the use of our legs, this does not mean that we do not have brains," a politicized statement complemented by her faith in God. Second, Firouzeh exercised ingenuity in drawing upon local resources. For example, when she had to take her children to the doctor, she would call a taxi and ask the driver to put her wheelchair in the trunk. When she took the bus, "I would ask some nice guys to carry my wheelchair into the bus and out again."

Firouzeh's use of the wheelchair as a stroller, her extended use of the taxi (to include her wheelchair) and seeking help from "the nice guys" to manoeuvre travel show her creativity and resourcefulness to get around and thereby use public spaces that would otherwise be inaccessible to her. For Firouzeh, home in her country of origin was a complicated affair. She left her natal home so as not to be a burden on her family. When she got married, she directed her efforts towards exploring and using public spaces in ways that were an extension of her home. Supported by her husband's waged work, she assumed the role of a mother and a wife. She refused to wear the label of disability as the sole marker of her identity, subverting the notion that "disabled" parents cannot raise children.

Disrupted Home-Life

Firouzeh's home-life, which she described as beautiful, was disrupted when Hossein joined a paralympics tour that brought him to Canada, where he claimed refugee status. He had hoped that his wife and children would be able to join him within a brief period. This did not happen because he experienced difficulties in getting a job. The couple was united only eight years later. When Firouzeh came to Canada with her children, she discovered that Hossein did not have a "home." She sensed it at the airport, a defining moment, considering their long separation. Her expectation was, "my husband would meet me at the airport with a bouquet of flowers. We were separated for eight years." Also, she observed that he did not kiss her or hug her. When she went to the place where he lived, she discovered that he had a simple life, that is, the bare minimum. He slept on a single bed that he had made himself; other items included a small dining table, a few plates, and some cutlery. She was disappointed as she had heard that persons with disabilities were well looked after in Canada. And Hossein did not have a job, though he had tried hard to find one.

Firouzeh relayed that the very next day she cleaned the house and made breakfast. This was the starting point for re-making her home. The family stayed in this place for three months after which Firouzeh followed up with BC Housing for a "family home." Being new to the country, she did not know how the system worked. She turned to her faith. "I promised Allah that I will say 14,000 *salwats*" (special prayers recited on beads). For two days, she said 13,000 salwats and held 1,000 back. The second day, in the afternoon, she got a call that BC Housing had found her a place. Once the family moved in, she recited the rest of the salwats.

Firouzeh's task of re-making a home was rendered more difficult because Hossein had become bitter and angry that Canada had not offered him opportunities to make a life for himself and his family. This had to do with the fact that he was "written off" as unemployable: his perceived "disability" and race (the Other) worked against him. In the wake of these circumstances, Firouzeh decided to take up the challenge of re-making a home for the family. She highlighted four narrative moments that demonstrated the meaning that home assumed for her in her county of settlement.

The Wheelchair Incident

> They take forever to give me any kind of service. For example, once my wheelchair did not work. It took two weeks. I sat on the sofa for two weeks. I phoned the company and asked. They said "our workers are not here, and they are on vacation. They will come later." When they came to take the wheelchair and repair it, it took two weeks. I could not go to school during that time. I could not get any work done. I just went to the bathroom every night and then slept the rest of the day. They should or could have lent me a wheelchair when they took mine away until mine is ready. In this way, a person would not be disabled from doing daily stuff. They must have the resources, but they do not want to do this.

Narrative scholars have informed us that people tell stories for two reasons: to make sense of their experience of suffering and to elicit a response from readers. Firouzeh, whose lifelong work consisted in re-making her world from scratch, is bent on drawing the reader's attention to an event that would otherwise be dismissed due to her social invisibility, along with the perception that refugees and immigrants should be grateful to be admitted to Canada. Firouzeh brings home the impact of her two-week confinement through her body language (sitting on the sofa) and subversion of the script: disability equals dependence.

In, *The Wounded Storyteller*, Frank (1995) informs us that the body does not speak, it begets speech. Firouzeh's portrayal of her body as being reduced to "nothing" (sleep all day) sends a powerful message to society. Her grounding of her body in space and time (on the sofa for two weeks) brings into relief her "suffering" that would otherwise remain unnoticed. The irony is well stated: while other people (the paradigmatic citizens) are on vacation, an immigrant woman with disabilities (a lesser being in the eyes of society) spends her time on the sofa. Note the effective use of dialogical strategy: "They said: 'Our workers are not here, and they are on vacation.'"

Firouzeh uses the wheelchair incident to show that she is not "dependent" and neither is she "disabled" in the way that society has constructed these social categories. Not having a wheelchair means that she is not able to perform her daily tasks, including attending ESL classes. Reconsider her words: *"They should or could have lent me a wheelchair when they take mine away until mine is ready. In this way, a person would not be disabled of doing daily stuff"* (emphasis added). This message reveals the workings of a disabling society. As Wendell has expressed it: "[D]isability is socially constructed through the failure or unwillingness to create ability among people who do not fit the physical and mental profile of 'paradigm' citizens" (1996, 41).

Taking a Bus

Firouzeh uses the bus to go to places even when there is an emergency. Her experiences with bus drivers have generally not been pleasant. She has been dismissed as an unworthy commuter.

> Most of the bus drivers do not take you, some of them do. I have seen things. Most of the bus drivers are kind and human but some of them, because they do not feel like getting up from their seats and help a disabled person, they say wait take the next bus. But I have that time frame to get home and make dinner for my kids, as my kids have come back home so they need me. I have anxiety and stress and want to come home. The bus driver does not know how stressed I am, and the next bus causes me to be delayed by about two hours. I am late and am on the street for no reason. Yes, it has happened to me many times. The first year, I did not know anything. But now I have learned why this happens. The bus driver can take me on his bus. But he doesn't. I am a disabled person but I do everything on my own. I take care of myself. Even on the bus, I fasten my wheelchair on my own and fasten the seatbelt on my own. Even when I get off the bus, I push the seat in the same position as it was. So I do not let the driver get off the seat and do these things for me. I say: "I can do that." I do not want to bother others. Many disabled people cannot do that and really the bus driver should help them. I am very careful with these things, not to be a burden on the driver.

When the bus driver stops to pick up passengers, he sees a "brown" woman sitting in a wheelchair. During his training, the bus driver would have received instructions on inclusiveness, yet is likely to perceive Firouzeh's "disabled" and racialized body as being of lesser value, due to societal attitudes towards the Other. We must note that this is not the case across the board. Race and gender-based discrimination must not be assumed. They are enacted in everyday life situations.

In retelling the bus driver incident, Firouzeh begins with the testimonial genre of "you." In doing so, she brings the reader into her space. In other words, it is only after she has secured an audience/an attentive ear that she tells her story. Not wanting to present herself as a victim, she begins with positive words, "most of the drivers are kind and human." This statement brings home the impact of unkind actions. This play of words serves her well. By not stereotyping all bus drivers as racist, her lived reality achieves more credibility.

Firouzeh highlights a second point. She states that the bus driver's reluctance to take her on board would mean that he must put in more work. He has to get up from his seat, lower the front seat to make room for her wheelchair, and fasten a seat belt around her. Firouzeh explains that he does not have to do any work. "I am a 'disabled' person but I do everything on my own. I take care of myself." This includes fastening her seat belt and, more important, putting the bus seat back to its original position. She notes that the bus driver's refusal to take her on board prevents her from preparing dinner for her children in good time. In the eyes of society, she is an immigrant woman with disabilities. Her self-inscribed identity is that of a mother and a wife, someone who runs a home like every other woman. She also attends classes. Firouzeh uses the bus incident to bring home the point that she is a functional human being, and is reclaiming a humanity that society has denied her.

A couple must not be seen in wheelchairs

Hossein is conscious of the image of "The Wheelchair Couple" after twenty-seven years of marriage. Hossein's discomfort is a function of compounded factors: racialized persons with disabilities being socially excluded along with a discriminatory immigration policy. Racialized persons are often asked the question: "Where are you from?" and racialized persons with disabilities are given the societal message: "You should not be here as you are a drain on our system." Immigration policy excludes this constituency, rendering them socially invisible. When in the public sphere, Hossein and Firouzeh encounter people who are indifferent or racist. This does not rule out individual acts of kindness and compassion. Being excluded from society, however, means that they are at the mercy of other people, who may be either insensitive or kind. Hossein's and Firouzeh's experiences in their new homeland in Canada have largely been negative. While Firouzeh is a fighter, Hossein harbours anger and frustration that has built up over eight years. When he first came to Canada, he wanted to work. But waged work was ruled out because he was judged unfit "just because I am 'disabled.'" Alone and isolated, he went through a prolonged period of depression. When Firouzeh joined him, he became more conscious of the couple's disability because it was fostered by a disabling environment. Hossein's experiences of exclusion are so acute that he sees his own wife as "disabled" rather than as the mother of his four children.

The above context explains the marital abuse that Firouzeh was subject to at the time of the study. On one occasion, she asked for professional help.

> I had a problem with my husband, a disagreement about something. I phoned and asked for help, so a worker came in. I phoned, and I said, "I do not know English and I need a translator. I have problem with my husband and I need help." They suggested to come and take me away from my home if the problem was too harsh. They said, "we can take you to some home until the problem is solved." I said "no, my problem is not that bad that you take me somewhere else. You can come as a friend, as a worker, as a leader or as an advisor to talk to both myself and my husband. Talk to my kids so that we can find a solution. I do not like to separate from my husband. That would not be good for my kids. Not good for me or my husband. You can come here and talk to all of us."
>
> We made an appointment and two Canadian workers came in and talked in two sessions with my husband and myself with the help of a translator. And it helped. Later, my husband was supposed to phone again and ask for an appointment. But he did not. And they did not come back. But they did not even check with me to ask if I still have a need or not, if I still have a problem or not. And later, I went to see those workers in the organization that they work. I wanted to talk to them. But I was told that they are not there or were on vacation, so up to now I have not been able to tell the workers how I feel.

Domestic abuse of racialized immigrant women is not merely a result of culture, as common perception has it. It is a function of these women's subordinate position in Canadian society. Their vulnerability is accentuated by unresponsive and insensitive social and health systems. What is overlooked here is that immigrant women, including those who are "disabled," are disadvantaged on multiple fronts. They are given low priority for job training and ESL classes, they are underemployed or unemployed, they face a double workload, they are socially isolated, and they are exposed to discrimination and racism in their daily lives. When they seek health or social services, they face barriers of language and access to services, as noted earlier. This scenario amounts to living within an unresponsive environment. Yet stories offer a medium for individuals to reconstitute themselves and find some way out, however minuscule it may be.

When Firouzeh phoned her social worker, she laid out the parameters for the kind of help that she required: a translator and family counselling. Her worker suggested that she move into a women's shelter; she did not consider Firouzeh's need to keep the family together. Nurturing her family was a lifelong labour that helped to reverse an all-encompassing disability identity. Firouzeh further suggested a model of "care" that blurred the boundaries between friend/worker/leader/advisor. This alternative mode is worth considering in light of the relatively linear and one-size-fits-all approach of professional social workers. As Ong argues (1995), professionals are made to do the policing work of the state. This includes controlling the body of the Other, a task carried out through the medium of the Eurocentric biomedical model. In Firouzeh's case, the social workers offered two sessions for the complex and painful experience of marital abuse. Furthermore, they left it to the husband – the perpetrator – to follow up. Firouzeh is acutely aware that she has not been served well. "They did not even check with me to see if I needed help and if I still have the problem." Upon her visit to the office, she was informed that the workers were busy or on vacation. Inaccessibility and lack of services constitute forms of control.

Firouzeh advances several points. Despite her language limitations, she lays out the parameters of her "therapy." She rejects the individualized model in favour of family therapy. Second, she criticizes the system for its indifference. In the process, she reinforces a point made by feminist scholars that women's social and health needs are consistently overlooked in a male-dominated society (Lee 1999). These needs are further dismissed in a racialized society. Firouzeh's visit to the office is a pragmatic move filled with some hope that she might come across a responsive soul. But this is not the case. Her message to society (the listening audience) is effectively conveyed: "I wanted to *talk* to them but I was told that they are not there or were on vacation." Firouzeh's portrayal of the image of a woman being turned back from a place that has an obligation to help says it all.

My Kids Are Hungry

People who receive social assistance have a difficult time. They are constantly reminded of the fact that what they receive is charity and not an entitlement. Overlooked is the fact that people's desire to undertake waged work is thwarted by an indifferent society. Firouzeh wanted to work. "I am not the type of person who isolates herself and says, 'I cannot do anything.' I like to participate in the community. I may have lost my legs, but I can use my brain, my hands, my eyes, my ears, my fingers. *I still have these*" (emphasis in the original). She is an active woman who happens to *use* a wheel-chair as opposed to being wheelchair bound.

About a month ago, I had a problem. We had nothing at home. No food and no money to buy food. We had run out of money, and my husband did not let me tell anyone about this. Maybe some one could give us a small amount of money or help me somehow. But he would not let me tell anyone. I phoned a lady I know and I told her that we did not have anything at home. I do not know what to do. She told me to go to my financial worker and tell her that I do not have groceries at home and my kids are in need of food. See what the worker can do for you.

I went to the office of that financial worker. There was a lady. She was a new worker. She did not know me. I told her my name and my husband's name and introduced myself. I told her that we are a family and I said that we have not had any grocery for one week. She said: "We cannot help you or give you something." I was sad and told her, "What should I do now? My kids are hungry and need food." She said: "You should use the disability benefits you have, and spend it in a way that you do not run out of money in the middle of the month." I know that. We are four people to live on $1200. From this $300 goes for the rent in addition to what the government pays. It is hard and then we have other bills.

She started telling me how I should spend the money. I became very upset and started crying. I said: "I came here with hope and now you are talking to me like this." Then I dialed my friend's number on my cell and let her talk to the worker in English. So she told the worker to help me somehow so Firouzeh does not get embarrassed when she goes home. So the worker said, "I can give you $80 to spend on grocery, and then we can deduct it from your next month's check." I went to an Iranian supermarket and bought food and vegetables. When my sons came home from school, they were happy and they told me: "How good that we have something to eat after two weeks." They said: "Thank you Mom and kissed me on the cheek." I told them that I got the money from my worker. Anyhow, she helped me but that was not easy to get the help. It was hard. The food lasted until the next cheque came.

Firouzeh begins her story on a temporal note. By stating that the incident occurred a month ago, she imparts continuity to her story. This was one moment among others that constitute part of her everyday life. The past is present. It cannot be dismissed as a bygone incident until it is rectified structurally. Second, Firouzeh introduces a human dimension, despite the crisis. "I told her my name and my husband's name and introduced myself. I told her that we are a family and ... that we have not had any grocery for one week." Although she barely speaks English and had no translation services, she conveys her message loud and clear: namely, that her family with two children had not eaten for one week. When Firouzeh secures $80, to be deducted from her next payment, she makes it a celebration. She shops at an Iranian food store, cooks, and serves the meal without letting her children or her husband know the difficult time she had in getting the money. She just says: "I got the money from my worker." But at the same time, she responds to the patronizing worker. "The food lasted until the next cheque came." She leaves it to the imagination of the reader to fill in the blanks, including her resourcefulness in stretching the $80 groceries for two weeks, feeding four mouths.

Re-making a home for Firouzeh entails drawing in entitlements from the public space, an aspect that does not come into play in a world where the demarcation between the private sphere of the home and the public sphere of the marketplace is sharp.[4] It is within the wider expanse of the home that Firouzeh seeks to address the issue of the conjoined unit of the private and the public and, by extension, life and death. I am reminded of Lambek's (2016) observation, "Death is a centrality of life, ostensibly the opposite of life, but also its very condition" (630). By subverting the notion of a self-sufficient subject, Firouzeh positions herself to speak to the tension between the fragility of life and hope for its rejuvenation, even in death. One cannot assume that death is the end of life. As Lambek had noted, What is it that dies in the event of death and what is it that lives?" (ibid.). It is this question, among others, that will be Firouzeh's legacy for her children, who take pride in her accomplishments under trying circumstances. It would be a legacy of survival, uncertainties, and hope against all odds. Such a legacy can form part of the repertoire of societal understanding of life and death, each being a condition of the other. Its realization requires rescripting neighbourhoods so that when people like Firouzeh seek entitlements, as opposed to charity, they encounter more humane forms of being where their personhood is recognized relationally. Death is forever present in life. It is in this context of relationality that one can strive to establish the parameters of social palliation.

Firouzeh adopts the socially valorized roles of a mother and a wife to define herself as a woman in the wake of society's rejection of her body and therefore of her personhood. She raises four children with pride and a sense of accomplishment. In doing so, she reclaims her humanity. This is one aspect of her storied life. In her own way, Firouzeh is effecting a paradigm shift towards social palliation, which is referred to differently by scholars seeking to promote transformative change. In

A Passion for Society, Wilkinson and Kleinman (2016) refer to it "as the enactment of substantive human values and as a moral commitment to building humane forms of society" (xi). Mattingly (2010) reminds us to be attentive to "moments of possibility and community that are cultivated and cherished across formidable divides" (3). She highlights two points that resonate with Firouzeh's story. First, despite tremendous odds, ordinary people exercise subjectivity in everyday life. Second, their struggles "to remake lives in the most remarkably barren social circumstances" (4) can bring about progressive change. Towards this end, Zarina and Tamiza (chapter 5) shared their stories not merely to relay their lives but also to make a difference for the larger society, a difference that I have referred to as social palliation, as opposed to palliative care.[5]

Homa's and Firouzeh's narratives take us to the threshold of human vulnerability and susceptibility, transforming our thinking of a bounded and discrete home where suffering is rendered invisible. Both women are animated persons wishing to share everyday enactments embedded in social and bodily know-how. These practices are analogous to affect, imagination, and intuition rather than rationalization. It is in this vein that both women reveal the vitality of human experiences that shape the multiple and contradictory positions that marginalized subjects occupy. In their own ways, these women question existing ways of apprehending the world; in the process they reveal the contours of social palliation, which translates into small acts of caring.

5 Negotiating Deep Divides: Foregrounding Social Palliation

Tamiza is the mother of two children, one of whom has been diagnosed as autistic, the other as hydrocephalic. In telling her story of raising them in a society that continues to segregate and stigmatize persons with a disability, Tamiza exemplifies a perspective captured by Yee: "But we know the issues that face us because we have lived them, they are our lives" (1993, 4). Tamiza's story is of interest because of how she reflects on her everyday experiences of negotiating the deep divides between the biological and the social, the private and the public, Us and the Other, all of which speak to the question of "home," its opening up into a world of social relationships, along with the question that I reiterate: "What are the factors that compromise our humanity and how it can be restored in social palliation?" The larger anthropological question echoed by Das and Han (2016), Fassin (2010), and Garica (2010) is: How do we confront the realities of human life as being finite and fragile and "what is it for a human being to be awakened to his or her existence"? (Das and Han 2016, 3). Acting and reflecting (praxis) on this question constitute the axis of Tamiza's testimonial narrative. Here, self-representation is rendered into "re-presentation of an experienced embodied social reality" (Bannerji 1995, 12), which for Tamiza constitutes a critique of the divides noted above.

As researchers, we are often tempted to rework the chronology of events framed by a narrator. But in such a process we risk overlooking the nuances and subtleties built into the narrative structure. For this reason, I have remained close to Tamiza's own account. I have also exercised caution so as not to suggest that she speaks from the discrete space of a racialized mother – a space to which minorities are often relegated, indicating that they can only comment on their own issues, and not those of the larger society. Like Firouzeh, Tamiza seeks to effect a paradigm shift towards social palliation, a caring society.

In the wake of deep listening, I anchor Tamiza's story into a larger socio-political context. My goal is to show that the issues she discusses and brings home are not only applicable to her story on "how I raised two children."[1] This is the world where life and death are folded into each other, a perspective that comes to life when we open the space for "ethics of care," as Garcia expresses it (2010, 209). Here, the concern is "not just what constitutes life, but what constitutes livable life" (Shaw 2018, 43) or "a good life" (Arendt 1958; Boehm 2008; Constable 2014). A good life, I argue, is not lived in isolation. It is relational, where both life and its underpinning of death assume existential significance.

Points of Entry: Reading Her Narrative

The birth of a baby can be a joyous occasion, and this was Tamiza's experience. "Faizal's birth brought a lot of joy and happiness. We were so happy that I decided to have a second child right away." Tamiza recalled that her son was toilet-trained and walking by the time he was one year old. "But I knew that something was wrong. I was constantly comparing him with my sister's son." Tamiza observed that Faizal was not learning and following directions like her nephew. She took him to a pediatrician and he informed her that everything was fine; all that she had to do was give him some time, because boys are slow. When Faizal was placed in a day care, his teacher put him into a special program. "They took my child and kept him with mentally retarded children. I had never been exposed to disabled children before. I said: 'My child does not belong here. My child can walk and talk. If you can't provide the service, I will take him somewhere else.' I was so hurt that Faizal was thrown with other mentally retarded children. We took Faizal to a specialist and he said that my son is autistic."

Tamiza came to Canada in 1976 with desirable social capital. Her fluency in English and a BA degree meant a deceptively easy entry into the job market. But she occupied the lower sector of the labour force, reserved for immigrant women (Agnew 1996). "I found a job the next day." Tamiza worked at two jobs: as a bank teller and as an evening babysitter. Within two years, she got married. The couple had two children, both of whom were diagnosed as "disabled." Tamiza related that she was fortunate to have family support. Her major struggle, highlighted in the narrative in different contexts, was to secure social services and to ensure that her children were recognized as persons who were just different. From her vantage point as a marginalized woman of colour, Tamiza identified two challenges: unfamiliarity with the social service system and inaccessibility. "I think it is wrong to keep these services [mainstream] 'hidden.' I let the others [minority women] know that these services are there. It is their *right* to use them" (emphasis in the original). Tamiza made a clear distinction between mainstream and minority populations. She considers the latter to be more disadvantaged and "therefore it was hard for me to find out what services were available. Even then, I had to struggle to get these services."

Narrative Moments

How I raised my children

Tamiza's first son, Faizal, was diagnosed as autistic. This condition is defined as "a complex developmental disability that typically appears during the first three years of life" (Autism Society of America 2000, 2; also Waltz 2005). The society's web-based write-up explains how autism as a *disorder* makes it hard for autistic people "to communicate with others and relate to the outside world" (ibid.). The reader is informed about the possibility of aggressive and self-injurious behaviour along with the fact that people with autism may also exhibit unusual responses to people and resist change. A biomedical focus is evident in the discourse of individual deficit: "disorder," "aggressive," "self-injurious behaviour," and so on. The section, "What are People with Autism Like?" highlights further disorders, such as "lack of spontaneous or imaginative play." Under the heading "Effective Approaches," we learn that early intervention is the best solution to the "problems" associated with autism. Autism as an abnormal condition that requires professional intervention is the sole focus of the article. The article's authoritarian, all-knowing approach leaves little room for the experiential and embodied knowledge of people who are autistic or those who care for them. We are not questioning the benefits of early intervention, but the focus on disease/defect/abnormal discourse is dehumanizing. The article makes no reference to the message that people with disabilities have spelled out loud and clear: "We are not defective beings but people who are different." Its emphasis on disembodiment (a universal autistic person) erases differences of race and gender, both of which require consideration, as they constitute the axis of social inequality.

Tamiza takes issue with the deficiency discourse on autism as an exclusively neurological disorder. "He (Faizal) is high functioning and verbal. He can talk and he can let his needs be known. Most of the autistic children that I have encountered are non-verbal." Tamiza's focus on the lived reality of her son comes out in other scenarios, most notably in her articulation of him "being a Muslim" and "being a Canadian" with citizenship rights.

> He is a volunteer. He picks up all the garbage and distributes flyers. He also helps with other things. He has learned a lot from the community and the community has learned from him. If I keep him in the closet like some other parents do, *the community will never learn, they will never learn* [emphasis in the original]. Faizal has taught the community so much. For example, when it comes to distribution of ritual food, everyone is supposed to take one. If someone asks for two, he says it loudly: "You are not supposed to take two." No one can dare ask for two when Faizal is around" [the mosque].

Tamiza portrays her son as active in the community. Her emphasis on mutual learning flies in the face of the dominant discourse focused on medicalization and the dependency status of people with disabilities. More important, her speaking about her son's activity, otherwise unnoticed, suggests the enactment of a different kind of citizenship, which Das and Addlakha refer to as "publics constituted through voice" (2001, 512). The issue is that what is otherwise constituted as private, such as the domestic sphere or a place of worship, is politicized in a way that leads to a paradigmatic shift. Here, disability and impairment are located "not in (or only in) individual bodies, but rather as "off" the body of the individual and within a network of social and kin relationships" (ibid.). Following Das and Addlakha, I argue that sociality, however tenuous, makes it possible for a person with disabilities to claim her/his citizenship in all kinds of dispersed sites. This potential is brought to light in the second vignette.

> You know I do not "hide" my children. When people ask me, I tell them that they are "special needs" children. If they do not understand, it is their problem, not my problem. I tell Faizal that he should use Islamic words, *al hamdulillah* [everything is due to Allah] and *sukhran lillah* [I am grateful to Allah], all the time. His workers [caregivers] ask what this means and this way they learn more about Islam.

Affirming a Muslim identity means being part of the global *Umma* (Islamic community) whereby one lives within and outside national boundaries, in other words, transnationally. We may note that nation-states do not promote deterritorized and borderland positions. Pluralism is antithetical to a postcolonial imagining of a nation-state. The latter is "a regime of order and knowledge" (Malkki 1995, 4) instituted to maintain the power and hegemony of one group to the exclusion of others. Yet cracks and ruptures appear in this imagined landscape, giving rise to alternative discourses and imaginings. A case in point comes from a community of British Pakistani Muslims. In a study of this community in Bradford, UK, Bagguley and Hussain (2005) comment on the second generation of Muslims' use of St George's flag to claim their identity as British Muslims during the 1998 World Cup. While the flag served "as a symbol of their belonging within and support for England" (213), it was always in conjunction with their global identity as Muslims, Pakistanis, and beyond. The contradictions and ambivalence that racialized minorities encounter in the West are not lost on the authors. They note that these British Muslims did not endorse the Union Jack, as it "is seen as a racist flag, the symbol of colonialism" (216). Yet their adoption of St George's flag is ironic, because it represents the crusades against Islam. Such is the nature of the in-between spaces where minorities lay claim to substantive citizenship and belonging.

Faizal lives in a group home. Tamiza stated that this is the best situation for him because he can participate in various activities. "He is so busy that I can only reach him in the evenings." Tamiza also wants to ensure that Faizal grows up as a Canadian Muslim. She is painfully aware of the fact that the group home is a mainstream institution. It does not cater to the cultural or religious needs of the multicultural population. Tamiza stated that Faizal gets exposure to his culture and faith, and his community during the weekends, when he goes home and she takes him to the mosque. By ensuring that Faizal prays every day in the group home and that he uses Islamic words during his interactions with (mainstream) service providers, she has carved out a space where Faizal is able to express his identity as a Canadian Muslim.

To assert an Islamic identity in the public sphere post-9/11 is no mean task. Tariq Modood's (2005) comments are relevant to Muslims living in the West: "They [the Muslims] have found themselves bearing the brunt of a new wave of suspicion and hostility, and strongly voiced if imprecise doubts are being cast on their loyalty as British citizens" (viii). Ironically, Faizal can speak as a Muslim and lay claim to public space, however limited, because, in Tamiza's words: "He is innocent. He cannot hurt anyone." The context for this remark is the increasing surveillance and policing of Muslims in the West post-9/11 (Thobani 2007). Faizal's practice of Islam (he also says his prayers in the evenings) establishes his presence in a group home in Canada. This is a significant step given the fact that "Muslim groups and the strategies they articulate for claiming rights to citizenship encounter particularly intense resistances and become the subject of intense scrutiny" (Isin and

Siemiatycki 2002, 191). The claim that Muslims make to assert their citizenship rights is a challenge. It entails rethinking "the universal figure of 'western man' as the universal bearer of citizenship rights and obligations, just as other social movements have called into question the male, heterosexual, white, able-bodied, and propertied man as the universal exemplar of citizenship rights" (ibid., 208). In the wake of increasing racial profiling of Muslims and further interrogations of whether Islam is compatible with western liberal democracy, Faizal's everyday enactment in a public space (Islamic greetings and prayers) must not be dismissed lightly. It may be understood as an act of intervention, suggesting another way of being that ultimately comes down to reaching out and claiming a space of belonging, leading to social palliation. His mother has trained him to express himself as a Muslim-Canadian. Claiming this identity in a public space is a step towards securing his rights as a citizen whose relationship to the nation-state is complex. This point is brought home by Tamiza's observation: "I want my son to be a good human being in this world," which she qualifies as "a good Canadian-Muslim." The issue here is that racialized people with disabilities are claiming a multi-layered identity; it is within this complex sphere that their ascribed status of disability as an absolute marker is subverted.

To explore this process of alterity and becoming, I present narrative moments from everyday life. This vantage point allows us to link local scenarios to structural and institutional complexes without diluting people's lived realities.

Disability as Tragedy

> At the time we were coping with my first son, I was already pregnant. At this time, I was seeing a gynecologist. We had to pay $500 extra for this service. When I did not hear from the doctor, I phoned him. There was no reply. I phoned again and asked the secretary why the doctor was not getting back to me. She told me that there was something seriously wrong with the baby that I was carrying. But she would not tell me. I told her that I wanted to know. She said that it was Chinese New Year and that the doctor is not available. I said: "I am coming there right now." I phoned my husband at work and I told him that there was something wrong with the baby that I was carrying. He came right away. When we saw the doctor, he said, "Your son has hydrocephalus," and he left the room. We had never heard of this word before. My husband said, "Let us go to the library." We did some research and found out as much as we could. We phoned my brother who is a doctor. He told us that if he has hydrocephalus, we are going to have a lot of problems. I said: "I don't want this baby. I cannot take

care of two disabled children." I was six months pregnant and it is illegal to have an abortion at this time. But there was a doctor who was willing to perform an abortion. I did not sleep the whole night. In the morning, I told my husband that I want this baby. My husband was very supportive. He is my best friend. I am ashamed that I was considering aborting my baby.

This account brings home a poignant issue: the tension between the desire to raise a child with a disability and societal pressure not to bring such children into the world. It is this scenario that explains why Tamiza considered aborting the fetus. The actions of the three medical practitioners are revealing. The first one walked out of the room, dismissing the unborn life through body language, while the second focused on the problems of raising a child with hydrocephalus. The third doctor's willingness to perform a late and therefore an illegal abortion speaks for itself. Strangely, the indifferent gynecologist and the "sympathetic" doctor both give the same message: it is not desirable to bring a child with disabilities into the world. Disability-as-tragedy is a view perpetuated in genetic screening.

It takes considerable theoretical agility to urge the public to support screening programs to prevent the conception of handicapped individuals while at the same time insisting that full respect be paid to such developmentally disabled adults that are already among us. (Reinders 2000, 1; also see Lock 2007)

There is a profound contradiction in this scenario: we cannot take the lives of the unborn (read "defective" fetuses), and at the same time respect people among us with disabilities. People with disabilities are reminded of their socially constructed abnormality in everyday life situations within neighbourhoods, workplaces, and social and medical institutions. But these situations do not preclude human agency. People on the margins challenge "the dominating centre by creating a public space and employing empowering poetics of the periphery" (Cheungsatiansup 2001, 32). In niches and crevices within dominant systems, persons with disabilities re-make their worlds, affirming their worth and value as human beings. Tamiza's decision to give birth to her baby is a commitment to bring the above script to the fore: disability = difference = valuable.

When I was pregnant with Ayaz, I was monitored every week. At the same time Faizal was going through tests. So, I was struggling with two things at the same time. When I was seven months pregnant, the doctors had to drain the fluid from Ayaz's brain as they were scared that his eyes would be affected. I had a C-section at seven months. When they delivered the baby, I did not see him for five months. When I held my baby the first time it was very hard. He was in the hospital for a long time. He had a couple of surgeries as they had to make sure that his optic nerve was not damaged by the fluid in the brain. There was one thing after the other.

Monitoring, surgery, eyes, fluid, optic nerve, brain – these are corporeal words. Here, the body is subject to what medical anthropologists refer to as "the scientific tradition of reductionism." This tradition assumes that to understand "the properties of the whole, we must first consider the units that compose the whole" (Lock 1993, 370). Such an approach dismisses experiential knowledge as irrelevant. Cultural influences of all kinds are viewed as getting in the way of revealing relevant facts "in the depths of the body" (ibid.). Lock takes issue with this in two ways. First, she argues that medical knowledge, while of value, is partial and fragmentary and rests on an abstract plane unconnected to time and space. "A person however, is clearly not an abstract entity, but a conscious being perpetually in a state of change, whose body is the centre of ongoing dynamic interactions among physical and social surroundings" (ibid., 371). Second, our body insists on meaning rather than existing as a surface to which things are done. The emphasis here is on the body as an active agent, whose engagement with the world does not exclude "the very sinew, nerves, and bones of the body" (ibid.).

The biomedical discourse that reduces her children to body parts ("fluid" and "optic nerve") is not what Tamiza accepts as her reality. Instead, she focuses on social relations.

How could I have rejected my own baby [considered abortion]. When Ayaz was born, both my husband's and my own family got together. I have a lot of support from my husband. We have become like friends. We laugh and cry together. We share our feelings. We have become very close. My mother quit her job to take care of Ayaz. Faizal was in the day care. But Ayaz needed a lot of care. His head was big. For three months he could not hold his head up and it was so big. I have been very lucky. The children have brought us a lot of happiness and joy.

Medical anthropologist Byron Good (1994) states that narratives provide avenues for relating and recounting, thus generating new questions and new perspectives. Tamiza's attempt to embed the family story into the biomedical frame is important because it provides her with the space and grounding to deal with the multiple issues that she faces as a mother of two "disabled" children. For Tamiza, family support gave her the anchor to venture into the outside world. "When I had so much family support, I knew that they were behind me and it was easier for me to explore what was out there."

Medical education at Harvard begins with *entry* into the human body, notes Good (1994, emphasis added). This stance is problematic because it trains medical students to look at the human body as an object to be skillfully manipulated. Good argues that the inward gaze into the body is out of step with the bodies that we interact with in our everyday life. Tamiza has embodied knowledge of this insight. In her account, she does not focus on the medical (read, compartmentalized and dehumanized) vocabulary. In our conversations, she emphatically observed that her children are contributing members of society. She notes that they have been instrumental in creating a special bond between her natal family and her in-laws, and between herself and her husband. She reiterates the point that her children have as much to teach the community as the community has to learn from them. This is a crucial point as, in the institutional context, people with disabilities are reduced to a population of service consumers who cannot give but only receive. This one-dimensional perspective erases the element of reciprocity, which is the bedrock of social palliation.

The demedicalized/alternative model is realized, not within the discrete entity of the individual body, but within *a network of relationships*. Reinders (2000), among others, argues that our social lives are in fact our moral lives, and our moral selves develop within the social relationships that we find ourselves to be part of. To accept responsibility for other people, we must regard our own lives in terms of those relationships (Das and Addlakha 2001). It is this aspect that is illustrated in Tamiza's account.

Advocacy work on the part of subordinate groups requires adopting a new subject position. This position is of interest because it goes beyond the individual unit that, in the Western philosophical tradition, is created out of the binaries of Self-Other and Subject-Object. Rather, this new subject is heterogeneous as well as political. "There are many narratives by women of colour around the world that propose and enact new forms of locating themselves within societies. These forms are both oppositional and non-essentialist, and they confront and fracture the self-other opposition in the name of inclusion, multiple identities, and diasporic subject positions" (Grewal and Kaplan 1994, 2; also see Dyck and Dossa 2007). Tamiza adopts multiple subject positions to advance the interests of her children,[2] always in the context of the larger society.

Multiple Subject Positions

Tamiza is constantly reminded of the multiple ways in which she and her children are excluded from social situations. Within her own community, she noted that she is not free to move around and socialize at events she attends with her younger son, a wheelchair user. She must wait for people to come to her. Likewise, she feels that people in general do not know how to approach her children. Their entry and exit points of interaction are confined to hello or how-are-you exchanges. It is interesting to note that Tamiza's narrative makes greater reference to service providers than people in her neighbourhood and the larger community; their absence is notable. Service providers tend to focus on instrumental and functional aspects rather than sociality (Dossa 2005; Kittay 2001). Tamiza seeks to rectify this situation, as illustrated below.

First, when Faizal graduated from high school, Tamiza had a party at her house. She invited people who interacted with Faizal daily: teachers, service provides, bus drivers, and classmates. "There were thirty people. Five of them were in wheelchairs. I had a barbecue and I served the food in my best chinaware. Why not these children should have fun like anyone else?"

Second, Tamiza uses the services of a nanny to help her take care of her children. Of interest is her emphasis on how "I treat my nanny as a family member. When we go out, I invite her." Tamiza has always had Filipino nannies because she thinks that they are reliable, and she feels at home with them. Tamiza stated that she has given her nannies (she has had several) time off so that they could upgrade their qualifications and settle down in Canada. "Even when they want to sponsor their families, I help them fill out the forms and give them letters of support."

Third, when Tamiza has to take time off from work to tend to her children, she lets her employer and co-workers know "the real reason. I can take sick leave and I don't have to let them know about my children. I am not going to hide my children."

These accounts emphasize one point. Tamiza wishes to establish her children's presence in the public sphere so they can be "heard" and "seen," a conclusion I draw from two questions: How are situations framed? What stories are circulated at moments in time and space?

Tamiza's desire to bring about change ("Why cannot disabled people get together and celebrate with non-disabled people?") is informed by the dominant discourse that renders people with disabilities as Other, especially those who are also racialized.

Tamiza was happy that I was interested in her story. She knew her children, like others diagnosed with disabilities, had been rendered

socially invisible. She related that when they visited places where people saw them often, they would greet them. But beyond that there was
no further interaction. "They [society] do not know how to address my
children. They do not realize that they are human beings like us. They
need to learn."

We should note that mainstream Canadians with disabilities also
struggle to access and secure services. Those who are educated are in
a better position to work their way around the bureaucracy. This also
applies to racialized minorities. Yet, according to Tamiza, the struggles
of minorities are greater for two reasons. First, no services have been put
into place for this population; their cultural traditions, along with their
structural exclusion, are not considered. Hence, they may not be able
to easily access the mainstream services they seek. Tamiza has therefore
taken it upon herself to spread the word within her own community.
Second, racialized minorities with disabilities face greater discrimination. To my question on racism, she said: "Yes, of course there is discrimination against coloured people and against Muslims. Right now,
I have to struggle for my children's rights to be human." Her stance on
acting as an advocate for all people with disabilities suggests that she
does not want to be confined to the scenario of "Let them fight their
own battles but they cannot speak for us [mainstream sector]." In other
words, she chooses to act as an advocate for all people with disabilities
to avoid a position where she is seen to be speaking exclusively for one
group. She continued,

> There are a lot of good programs inside this country and nobody is hand-
> ing them out. You must find out these programs and apply for these pro-
> grams and make sure that as a taxpayer it is your right. You should not be
> made to feel guilty that it is taxpayers' money. You should not be told that
> you should not be doing this [spending taxpayers' money]; you should be
> doing this on your own. You can't because there are a lot of major expenses
> you are looking at and you need assistance. You should not be ashamed to
> ask for it. But nobody is going to tell you for sure that "look this program
> is available and your child might be entitled for it."

Tamiza reiterates two intertwined issues: entitlement to programs
and inaccessibility of programs. She recognizes that some good programs are in place, but that people do not know they exist.

> I really worked for it. I have said it is not fair to dump a child on somebody
> and say it is your responsibility and you are on your own. I don't think
> it is fair. I think that the social worker or somebody else in social services

should come and sit with you and [tell you] what is available and what you need. And if you want to get in touch with us this is the way you apply for it. Because the parents go through so much, so much to deal with. The last thing they want is to worry. Apply for this home, fill up this application, go and see this person. You feel you are begging. They put a lot of stress on you. I want to give this message. There should be more information available to know what is out there.

The onus then is on consumers to identify the programs and secure them. "You just have to be aware and very assertive and just ask for them." The empirical issue of accessibility is linked to entitlements. Tamiza's experience indicates that she is made to feel guilty for using taxpayers' money, notwithstanding the fact that she worked for eight years before she had her children and that she returned to work after she found daycare for her children. She and her husband are both taxpayers.

Tamiza does not think that she is sitting back and relying upon services, though she considers this to be her right as a citizen and as a taxpayer. More important, she feels that she and her children are short-changed in social interactions. She noted that her children are actively engaged in programs that "are fantastic and keep them very busy. I have to wait until the evening before I can talk to them." But this is their world of doing (activities), not being. Referring to the latter, she gives the example of Faizal, who moves beyond the marker of "disability." "He does not allow me to park in the handicap spot when Ayaz is not with us, whether we are in the mosque or in a shopping mall." Faizal's refusal to wear an essentialized disability identity is telling. Priestley's (1999) work shows how children with disabilities, as social actors, "work out ways of placing themselves within and without the discursive categories of 'disability' and 'special need.' Rarely do these children use a reified category: disabled or non-disabled. They may assume disability identity to overcome societal barriers and once these are overcome, they switch over to other more flexible identities" (Priestley 1999, 99; also see Billington 2006).

Also, through Faizal, Tamiza gives her Muslim faith a public presence. She is motivated by one major factor. She believes that her heritage will impart an identity to her children that goes beyond that of disability as a master status. She believes her faith, anchored in history and oriented towards everyday life (through practice and embodiment), will give social recognition to her children. When Faizal observes his prayers in the evenings and invokes Islamic phrases during the day, he arouses the interest of the people around him. "Service providers often ask me what is the meaning of the phrase that Faizal uses. I explain to them in a straightforward way so that they understand." It means a lot to Tamiza that her children, in a small but incremental way, are making her religion visible. Anthropological insight into the importance of everyday events prompts me to situate Faizal's practice within a larger context, noted by Modood. "A hundred years ago the African-American theorist W.E.B. Du Bois predicted that the twentieth century would be the century of the colour line; today we seem to be set for the century of Islam-West line" (2005, 23). Tamiza's attempts to give a public presence to Islam and render it more inclusive creates new spaces where she can claim her children's humanity and those of others.

Advocating Alternative Ways of Being/Social Palliation[3]

The core issue addressed in this narrative is to show how Tamiza – a racialized woman caring for two children with disabilities – speaks to identify the fault lines of the system/social service sector and suggest avenues for change. Of interest is the narrative strategy that Tamiza uses to share her experiential knowledge of the system. We note that in the beginning she had no exposure to children with disabilities, a situation brought about by structural factors: the social invisibility of people with disabilities and an exclusionary immigration policy that does not recognize persons with disabilities as potential immigrants or wage earners. Early on, Tamiza discovered that she had to learn and negotiate the system on her own. She presents herself as a protagonist, a position that marginalized women adopt so that they can be heard, such is their silencing in society (Dossa 2004; Ross 2001). She is determined to know the system inside out, once she realizes that it is structured to remain out of the reach of people, especially those who are Othered. She notes, "Nobody, not even your doctor, will tell you that such and such a service is available. You have to find this out on your own." Tamiza spends a lot of energy and time to ensure that her children have the best of what is available; she acknowledges that her children were able to access the system because they started early in life. Other factors (ironic) at work were that both Faizal and Ayaz have well-defined medical diagnoses and that Tamiza is fluent in English. Being brought up in colonized Tanzania, she was able to familiarize herself with "how things work in the West."

Although Tamiza feels that she was able to secure services to her satisfaction, she is not content because of the fact that service provision comes with a price: services are given to her as charity and their task-oriented focus dehumanizes her children. Tamiza then wages a second battle: she presents herself and her husband as taxpayers, making the argument that services are entitlements. In terms of praxis (that is, she acts and reflects), she describes scenarios that address structural issues and contain political possibilities. The narrative moments reflect two themes: Tamiza's portrayal of her children as persons speaks to the fundamental premise of social palliation; here, personhood is recognized in the course of life and not at the end of life. Second, recognizing personhood calls for bridging private-public, medical-social, and East-West divides, critical components of social palliation.

In her narrative, Tamiza keeps the aspect of being human in the forefront. She takes issue with her sons having to adopt a totalizing disability identity to secure services. Tamiza brings home the point that task-oriented services (programs and activities) compromise the humanity of her children. They do things, but people are largely absent in their social landscape. By way of restorative/palliation work, Tamiza foregrounds the language of humanity and entitlements, complementing Fassin's (2010) and Stevenson's (2014) observations that life cannot be reduced to the biopolitical. Here, one's well-being is not just measured by what is needed to survive materially, "but what makes life worthy of being lived" (Jackson 2011, 60; cf. Shaw 2018, 44).

Tamiza shared the following extract through her email network – an extract that adds more strokes to the social palliation landscape.

I am the child who is mentally impaired

I don't learn easily, if you judge me by the world's measuring stick. What I do know is infinite joy in the simple things. I am not burdened as you are with the strife and conflicts of a more complicated life. My gift to you is to grant you the freedom to enjoy things as a child, to teach you how much your arms around me mean, to give you love. I give you the gift of simplicity.

Zarina: New Possibilities for Being and Belonging

Zarina was married to a wealthy family who lived in Kampala, Uganda. She came to Canada as a refugee during the Asian exodus. My first meeting with her took place in a yoga class organized by the Ismaili Seniors' Committee. While doing her own exercises, she was encouraging another woman (her friend) not to give up when the latter was finding it hard to lift her arms. When I asked her why she joined the class, she said, "We have to keep healthy otherwise who will take care of us. You know our children are busy." Having met her a couple of times in the class, she invited me to visit her at her home. When I arrived, she had prepared *chai nasta* (tea and snacks), noting, "I do not want to waste your time. You are doing important work. This is the reason I have kept everything ready, so we can begin right away." Seeing the album on the coffee table, I asked Zarina if she wished to comment on photos of her choice. Below is her account.

The first picture was that of Jamat Khana in Kampala. It is a towering structure that could be seen from any part of the city. Zarina observed, "This was my anchorage. I had a hard life in Kampala. Being married to a wealthy family was not easy. I had to live up to their reputation and status." She then showed me a couple of family photos. Her in-laws were seated in the centre, symbolizing their authority, as noted by Zarina. "Every morning, I had to go to my mother-in-law and ask her what I should cook on that day. She would give me a list of menu items, not realizing how much time some of the dishes required. I cooked for ten people; my husband's two unmarried sisters and two brothers also lived with us. I would be in the kitchen from morning till 1:00 p.m. when we had lunch. My father-in-law controlled the expenses. They were tight on money and I had to make do."

Flipping through the album, Zarina showed me the picture of her natal family. Dressed in a sari, she wore a broad smile and looked happy. She said, "This is the way of the world. You have a good life in your parents' home and not so happy life in the home of your in-laws. For me life was tolerable. This is because I went to Jamat Khana every-day with my children. I found peace in this place. I performed service (*seva*)." Other pictures Zarina showed me included extended family gatherings that she enjoyed. "I cooked a lot, but I liked interacting with my husband's family. Some of the aunts were nice to me and I got along well with them and others not so well. I like people."

When I asked Zarina to delineate her understanding of home, she said, "Home is where there are people. A place where you can occupy yourself. A place where you can have chai-nasta shared with people who drop in." She observed that life in Kampala was fine for her. It was not ideal, but she lived in a familiar environment. She could walk to Jamat Khana. She knew the streets near her home along with the people who lived there. Once or twice a week, she went shopping. She would meet other women on the way; she stopped and chatted with them. She also talked to the shopkeepers. Zarina enjoyed having visitors that she could interact with, but she dreaded the thought of doing all the work. "My mother-in-law did not help in the house. Her thinking was that *bahu* (daughter-in-law) should do all the work. When my own family visited, I had a 'holiday.' They would not allow me to do any work.

They would say, 'Put your feet up and rest. You will not be able to do this once we leave.' I liked having people as it was one way my three children (two girls and a boy) learnt about respect for elders, patience and service." When I asked her to give me examples, she shared imagery from the family's garden of fruit trees. "I would tell them to keep the image of a mango in mind. It needs time to ripen. Otherwise, it will not taste sweet [patience]. When it comes to respect, I would point to the trees and inform them they must be tended and nurtured as they provide shade to the people and shelter to the birds. I impressed on them the point that trees will always provide shade, regardless of how much exposure they have to the sun [trials and tribulations of life]."

When Zarina migrated to Canada, she left behind a familiar milieu. Her concern was not that of moving to another country but the absence of a people-oriented world where another person's humanity and personhood are affirmed. This is the aspect that she missed the most. "When I am out, no one greets me, not even neighbours. When you go to the store, it is as if you are there to just do your work: purchase what you need and then leave. It was not like this in my country. People talk to you and ask you how you are and how is your family."

Upon her migration, her son Rafique decided that his mother should live with him since his father had passed away in Uganda. He was married with two young children. Having his mother around was advantageous for him because she took care of the children and maintained the house. For the same reason, Zarina's older daughter also wished that her mother could have stayed with her. Being astute, with a sense of humour, Zarina noted, "Instead of being a grandmother, I have now become a grand caregiver, *cheh neh* (is it not?)." Based on the traditional norm of sons taking care of mothers (a norm that is no longer followed), the son had the priority; the issue is that both the children wanted their mother for babysitting and housework though Zarina mentioned that they did not spell this out. She could read between the lines. This does not mean that they did not love her.

Zarina stayed with her son and daughter-in-law for almost a decade, taking care of the children and cooking for the family. She observed that she felt isolated because during the day she was alone with the grandchildren. "No one dropped in. I missed not having people in the house." She relayed the point that her son and daughter-in-law had different schedules. She had to adjust to this situation as it was not unusual for them to eat at different times. The conversation at the table was kept at a minimum. There was not much that they shared with her. The outside world was deemed to be different as what counted there was work and performance with minimal space for affect. One scenario was telling, a scenario that I had the opportunity of observing during invitations at parties. "You know, my children respect me. They never tell me anything that would be perceived as negative. I still feel left out from their lives. All my children get together on many occasions. When it is time for dinner, they make me sit on the host chair, where my husband used to sit back at home. They all ask me how I am and if I need anything. They tell me to take good care of my health. Once this conversation has taken place, they talk among themselves about their work or events occurring in the outside world. I feel left out of this conversation. I sit there for the rest of the meal. I listen, but I do not feel included." On another occasion when I asked Zarina what TV programs she liked best, she said, "During the day time, I watch Indian programs. When my children come home, they want to watch *their* programs. In fact, when my children are watching their programs, like movies, I go to my room. If they are watching evening news, I stay for a while. What keeps me going is Jamat Khana. There is transport for seniors. I got to *Khane* (short form) every day."

Zarina welcomed my visits. I made it a point to see her whenever I could. Once when I went to her house, she was walking around with a cane. She said her legs were becoming unsteady and it was necessary for her to use the cane so that she could do some work and remain active. "I do not like to sit. This would make me feel that I am of no use. She cited an anecdote, "People who work are valued. Those who do not work become a burden." The latter was the state that she dreaded. Unfortunately, she fell down a couple of times and eventually became bedridden. That is when she decided that she did not wish to live. She talked little and ate little. After a year or so, she stopped eating, signalling that she desired to leave this world. It was during this time that she was admitted to a hospice where she was given water and boosters through an IV. According to her family, the doctor had indicated she would not live long. At one point, while she was still functional, I asked her to draw an image of the meaning of home for her. She drew three homes. The first one was from her country of birth. It was a big home with garden and stairs on which she drew people, indicating the flow of visitors. The second home was in Canada. Here, she placed the figure of a woman working inside the house – the figure representing herself. The third picture was that of a hospice. She drew a bed on which a person lay. The *gar* (home as opposed to the physical structure of a house) no longer existed for her. She decided she did not want to continue living. She placed emphasis on a bigger destination (*manjil*) where she would be united with her creator.

Although Zarina did not talk much about her own life in Canada, she highlighted a couple of scenarios that she thought reflected her and her cohort's predicaments. The first scenario concerns a woman, Noori, she had gone to school with. Noori lived in Vancouver while her two married sons lived in Ottawa and Toronto, respectively. Zarina observed, "Although I did not meet Noori that often, I knew that she was an active and an energetic woman. She was involved in voluntary work within our community and took care of her husband, who has Parkinson's. Furthermore, she maintained close ties with her five grandchildren. She would often travel to Ottawa and Toronto to spend time with them. She had impressed on them to say their prayers every day before going to bed. It so happened that Noori was diagnosed with terminal cancer and died within two months. Her children were left with the dilemma as to who would take care of the father. They came up with two options. The first one was to let the father live in the house that he had got used to with two caregivers, ensuring that one of them drove. The rationale was that this arrangement would allow the father to remain in a familiar environment. But the caregivers cannot take the place of family. The second option was to arrange for the father to live part-time with one son and part-time with another. 'O, my God, how could he keep on moving from one place to another.' This is what happens to us older people." Recalling the image of a tree, she observed, "they have forgotten that we provide 'the shade,' even when we are no longer in this world."

The second scenario she portrayed was that of her niece, who lost her husband through a massive heart attack. "Her three children (two sons and a daughter) live in Toronto. The children did not want the mother to live alone in Vancouver. They bought a condominium for her in Toronto near Jamat Khana. This way, they thought she could do service work (*seva*) in the Jamat Khana and occupy herself. They did not ask her if this is what she wanted. What would happen if her health failed her and she could no longer do seva? It is very sad that we are in this difficult (*mushkil*) situation. We cannot live with our children and we cannot live without them. Where should we live when we lose our *ghar* (home)?" At this point, Zarina recalled a verse from a ginan. "*Marana he ye jaroor, joog mahe cheti ne chalo*" (remember, we absolutely have to die, think how we can live righteously).

Zarina's narrative, along with the examples she cited, suggests this relationality and interconnectivity is lost in family and neighbourhood alike, a function of the neoliberal market economy, the impact of which is felt within the intimate spaces of everyday life.[4] Yet, in the course of my research, I discovered endurance and resilience in the women (and men) I was privileged to meet. They infused their everyday world with meaning while recognizing the vulnerability and fragility of life with its twofold dimension. The first is generic, in the sense that crises like illness and death are not uncommon experiences. As my participants reminded me, we are all going to die but we forget that this can occur anytime and during any period of life. Second, the vulnerability and fragility of life is exacerbated in the case of racialized minorities owing to their marginalized status. Citing the example of Canada, Razack (1998, 2008) argues that this country is imagined as white; this means that Indigenous people and racialized minorities will invariably be subject to structural exclusion. In a similar vein, Thobani (2007) observes that whiteness, which she refers to as "exalted subjects," has been the premise for nation-building in Canada. This scenario leaves no space for non-European people even though Canada is officially recognized as multicultural. We may note that in the post-911 era, Muslims have been vehemently targeted as the Other. This is because they are socially constructed as a security threat to advance the political agendas of countries in the West. Primarily, they are used as scapegoats to mask the fault lines of nation-states; rather than remaining silent, scholars have spoken up to present counter-narratives in the form of stories, discourse, practice, and activism (refer to Ghorashi and Moghissi (2010); Liebelt and Webner (2018); Said (1978); Selby and Beaman (2018); Thobani (2010); and Zein (2004, 2006, 2009). The burgeoning literature on Muslims and Islam barely discusses the role of these counter-narratives in social palliation. By way of a beginning, I present the following example from my fieldwork (April 2018).[5]

Sabrina

I came to know sixty-nine-year old Sabrina through a friend who suggested that I might wish to contact her because she had recently been diagnosed with terminal cancer. When I called Sabrina, I was informed by a close family member (Nargis) that she had been transferred to a hospice. Nargis informed me that Sabrina had visited a physician several times stating that she had severe back pain; she was given pain medication and encouraged to see a physiotherapist. But it was too late. She soon learned that she had stage four colon cancer. When I asked Nargis how Sabrina felt being misdiagnosed, she said: "Sabrina accepted her diagnoses gracefully. She did not blame the doctor for not having paid enough attention to her symptoms. She merely stated, "The time has come for me to go. My creator is calling me, and I must leave this world." Before I could visit her at the hospice, she passed away. Nargis gave me the following account.

> Sabrina informed her family, "The divine being has already held my hand (*aneh maro hath pakdi litho che*). I am going to die in peace." When she was admitted to hospice, she encouraged family members and her friends to visit her. She said, "whoever wants to visit me may do so. I do not have any reservations. I will gain from the prayers they will offer for me." Sabrina asked religious leaders to perform end-of-life ceremonies like that of forgiveness (*chanta*) and special prayers (*du'a*). Her family brought DVDs of her favourite ginans that were played as she wished. She talked to each family member conveying her wishes. For example, she told her grandchildren to always pray and never forsake their faith. "This is the only thing that will give you strength and courage," she would say. She asked her husband to continue with the service work (*seva*) that she performed within her community. She told her family members to go to Jamat Khana every day to the extent possible. In pieces of paper she wrote down special prayers that would help them during crisis. One morning at six o'clock, a nurse came to her room to take her pulse. She held her hand but could not tell whether she was sleeping or had passed away. She called another nurse and she confirmed that Sabrina had died; it was a very peaceful death.

Nargis enthusiastically speaking both loudly and softly shared the above account with me with the words, "You know, I have learnt a lot from her. I now know how to die peacefully." She added, "Everybody should learn from her. Good people like her die in peace." Nargis had no comment when I asked her about the hospice where Sabrina spent close to twenty days. My reading of the above vignette suggests that Sabrina had transformed her hospice room into a "home." She encouraged people to visit her. I learned that she loved it when they offered prayers for her. Those with a good voice sang ginans for her as well. Sabrina's hospice room was her spiritual space. This is where she recited daily prayers, obligatory for Muslims, and instructed her family how to follow the path of *sirat'ul mustakim* (the right path). While Sabrina's agency in the hospice may be considered singular, we need to foreground her work because it speaks to the core theme of this book: displacement, social wounding, and social palliation.

During my two later conversations/interviews with Nargis, I learned that Sabrina's story of displacement was no different from that of other participants. When she migrated from Kenya forty-two years ago, she and her husband had to start from "an empty space"; their credentials were not recognized. Sabrina was an elementary school teacher. She ended up working at a daycare as an assistant to a teacher (lower rungs of the ladder). She worked long hours, and sometimes worked in the evening. At the same time, she raised two children, ensuring that they became professionals: a nurse in the case of her daughter and an accountant in the case of her son. Their career paths required them to be mobile and they both left Vancouver, moving to other parts of Canada for better prospects. As Sabrina aged, she missed her children and grandchildren tremendously although they visited her when they could. To overcome her loneliness and isolation, she attended Jamat Khana regularly with her husband and engaged in service work. Sabrina's trajectory of life exemplifies the relationship between social wounding, displacement, and Islamic faith. Social wounding comes into play with the script of Otherness and structural exclusion. This is not the endpoint. The experience of being wounded suggests "returning the gaze," as Bannerji (1993) expresses it, whereby minorities carve a space for reconfiguring their lives in the wake of displacement. In the process, they draw upon a repertoire of traditions (dynamic sense), which in the context of this study is Islam. The latter is conceived not as static but as a lived and a palpable faith, which Sabrina activates by transforming the space of the hospice/palliative care into a "home-space," the significance of which can best be understood as potentially creating a language of understanding and engagement across socio-political boundaries (geopolitics from the bottom). This aspect informs the formation of social palliation.

In chapter 4 and this chapter, I have explored multiple ways in which participants re-make a home. Homa interrogates the boundary of nation-states, suggesting the formation of a transnational home; Firouzeh and Tamiza reinforce the point that home is not a discrete unit but is intricately connected to the public space. Zarina and her colleagues reveal the predicaments of re-making a home, suggesting that it is a partial undertaking; they bring to light the point that suffering is not devoid of endurance and re-making a life. Sabrina highlights faith-based elements for expanding the boundaries of a home within the space of a hospice. These protagonists bring into relief the importance of a new language for deep-level conversations (encapsulated in the sacred traditions) to effect a paradigm shift from palliative care to social palliation with its focus on existential moments of life and death. The social wounds they bear carry the seeds of new possibilities for being and belonging to the world where the implicit presence of religiosity must be recognized. As Jasmine Zine (2004) notes, Islamic faith-based epistemology presents another mode of being female in ways that disrupt Western secularism. She calls for a new discursive orientation from which Muslim women can locate their self-determined political and ideological projects to reclaim their autonomy (170). The participants in my study undertook this project in their own ways: through storytelling and sacred traditions, highlighting what it is like to live and what it is like to die in the contemporary age.

Conclusion

Sacred Traditions: A Forum for Deep-level Conversations

In this concluding chapter, I wish to create space for deep-level conversations through the prism of sacred traditions, with their emphasis
on primary symbols that speak to humanity. As a repertoire of knowledge on the foundation story of life and death, sacred traditions have
much to offer. I argue that the uncertainty and finitude of life can be
understood on the plane of social palliation where one's humanity –
what it is like to be a person in a conflicted world of inequality and
injustice – is not compromised. A critical point that I wish to emphasize is that the sacred is not confined to a discrete sphere. It exists
in a world of being and becoming that study participants sought to
restore after losing this milieu through displacement. This does not
mean that there were no issues in the participants' homeland. Speaking as wounded storytellers, they relayed their concern about loneliness and isolation in the country of their settlement; they felt that this
condition could be remedied through sociality and interconnectivity
(social palliation)[1] along with a sense of belonging that would allow
them to be in the world, reciprocally. It is within this realm, they
noted, that one can share the foundation story of humankind: what is
it like to live and what is it like to die. To illustrate this, I have organized this chapter as follows. In the first part, I summarize the two
narratives as I have understood them: those of the study participants
and those of the palliative care practitioners. I seek to demonstrate
that social palliation can bridge the spatial and temporal distances
that exist between the two groups. I include an overview of neoliberalism in the second part to identify the societal forces at work, forces
that compromise our humanity. In the third part, I present fragments
of the sacred traditions of the Canadian Ismaili-Muslims (South Asian
origins) and that of the Canadian-Iranians. I show how life and death
as a conjoined unit are articulated in these traditions. It is my hope

that the repertoire of this rich heritage will create space for deep-level conversations with other traditions, thereby effecting a shift towards social palliation.

Narrative Framing[2]

"Glimpses from the Stories of our Lives"

My interlocutors advanced the point that palliative care must not be confined to the clinical setting of a hospice, a designated area in the hospital, or a private home. They expressed reservations, noting that compassion and dignity of life are only proffered when one is nearing death. The questions they raised are: Should not the reality of life, with its trajectory of birth, growing old, and death be taken into consideration as a whole? Does an exclusive focus on death not amount to severing it from life? What about the circumstances of people who have crossed the border from a developing to a developed world? The divide between the two worlds has come about because of the militant colonization that has now been incorporated into neoliberal global capitalism. The latter, they would say, has disrupted their lives because the process of growing old has been severed from its life course of birth and death. With its emphasis on individualism and an autonomous way of being, neoliberal capitalism has undermined our lives, which were otherwise embedded within families and communities. Participants recalled scenarios such as "how once upon a time, we all lived together. Now we are dispersed. It is so sad that we do not have time for each other. How can this be possible that we cannot even interact meaningfully with our families and neighbours?" Continuing the conversation, they noted, palliative care is individualized, though we value what it has to offer: personal and compassionate care. Those of us who have crossed socio-cultural and geographical borders have alternative perspectives to offer but these are dismissed as not of much value. These perspectives are not given space in a society where our very lives are subjugated under the label of "racialized minorities," meaning the Other, not like us. At most, there is interest in our culture and/or our faith, but this focus can reinforce our Otherness because an exclusive cultural lens can separate and reify our lives even more. Allow me to present an example that is not atypical.

During my research, I came across families praying in unison for their loved ones in a hospice. Their prayers were heard by frontline staff who remained in the vicinity to assist in any way they could. The staff commented on the atmosphere of calm and peace generated by the recitation of prayers. In the words of a staff member named Karen, "I rarely experience this form of peace in my work. There was something special and unique that I gained by being here." The issue is that Karen did not have the space or the professional leeway to include these experiences in the system. The practices that the families enacted were confined to the space allocated to them. The question that the interlocutors posed was: How can we share what we know about dying and death (and life) with palliative care practitioners and through them with the larger society? This form of sharing would allow us to acquire a sense of belonging that is presently not the case because we are considered to be different. The interlocutors continued,

You may ask, how can we effect a paradigm shift from a clinically based palliative care to social palliation? Our response would be as follows. First, we have relayed the stories of our lives as we believe stories bring to light realities that cannot be expressed through other mediums. We have been subject to diasporic ruptures because our lives back at home were markedly different from our experiences in Canada. In our country, we had many issues that we did not always resolve. But we had family, social networks, and communities that we could turn to. We cannot do this anymore as we are uprooted from our homelands and our country of settlement is too individualized. Isolation and loneliness have become our companions, and this will affect how we will die. The neoliberal market economy considers older people to be redundant and a social burden even though in our younger years we contributed to the economic welfare of this country. It is our wish that our struggles to settle down and re-make a home under difficult circumstances are acknowledged not at the end of our lives but as part of who we are as persons. Social palliation, then, should form part of everyone's life as people go through their life trajectories (biological and social) and not just at the time of death. This is the insight we have shared through our life stories.

I recognize that what I have presented above is unconventional (my own summation of what I heard, observed, and witnessed). But it is necessary so as to provide a summary of my reading of the data. This may appear to be simplistic. It is not. These are insights that participants wish to share (engage into deep-level conversations, partially through deploying their sacred traditions) with palliative care practitioners, and, through them, with society and the world at large, a task that I seek to accomplish modestly through this chapter. It is only appropriate that we also hear what the practitioners have to say about their work. That is documented below in the same vein.

Narratives of Palliative Care Practitioners

If you were to ask palliative care practitioners to relay their narrative, this is what they would say: There are two things that you might want to know. First, palliative care has come about to correct the shortcomings of the biomedical model. It is standard practice for physicians to inform terminally ill patients that there is not much they can do for them. Upon realizing that there is no cure, physicians tend to withdraw from providing any form of care. This is where we come in. We say, we will take care of you until the moment of death. Our care is patient- and family-focused. This means that we will do our best to ensure that you and your family are comfortable and that the dignity of your life is maintained till the very end. We will ensure that your needs are given priority. The care we provide is compassionate and holistic. We support the family as well in every way, including bereavement. We have come a long way since palliative care became a subdiscipline within the medical field in the seventies. We emphasize the fact that a patient should get full attention from us not only physically but also socially and spiritually. A person should die whole. This means that we strive to develop communication skills that are unique to our field. We engage in active listening. We learn not to ask leading questions on medical interventions. We provide space to the patient and the family to make their own decisions. We seek an outcome that advances wellness and health; we do not focus on the sick person, the iconic figure in the medical establishment. We focus on who you are as a person. We take the position that no person should die alone and without compassionate care. We will hold your hand until the last minute because we believe there is life until the moment of death.

The issue we are grappling with is, How do we incorporate the cultural practices and/or faith traditions of minorities? We realize that this is challenging. We do not assume that we know what a culture is as we recognize that it is dynamic and therefore it must be understood contextually. Some of us take the view that we should adopt a case-by-case approach but then we also need to know generally what a particular culture and / or faith advocates when it comes to death. We have examples of how we have accommodated different minorities' culture and faith traditions. For instance, there was a Hindu woman who wanted to lie on the floor at the time of her death. We did not understand the reason, but we did not intervene. Later, her daughter told us that this was a way for her to detach herself from the material world. In a training session, an instructor put it this way, "We must learn, learn about what matters to them. We should understand what their concept of health and wellness is, understand what death means to them. If you do not know which particular group you are serving, your ability to do a good job is hampered." A practical approach is to ask questions on culture and religion as part of the admission profile. This way we can plant the seed, so to speak, for inclusive care.

Now that you have heard us, let us have a conversation about how we can bridge the two areas: your aspiration for social palliation and our limitations working within an institutional setting that we think we have transformed by introducing a compassionate form of care. The implications for this form of care should not be overlooked as it blurs the boundary between biological reality and social reality – a boundary that has remained intact within biomedicine.

Reader, I have presented two scenarios that seem to be miles apart. First, recipients and potential recipients of palliative care advocate a wider expanse where their lives are acknowledged, and their person-hood is affirmed in the course of living. They take the approach that clinical care is restrictive and the fact that it comes into play at the end-of-life is problematic existentially because it severs death from life. Practitioners take the approach that palliative care is invaluable because it restores dignity to a person at the end of his/her life – dignity, along with personal care that they do not enjoy in a hospital setting. Practitioners take pride in their work because they believe that their vision of holistic model of care restores humanity to a dying person.

Nevertheless, confining palliative care to a clinical setting limits the realization of its vision, the more so when it comes to addressing the concerns of racialized minorities. As noted in the introduction, the latter experience structural barriers because they do not have multidimensional access: materially, socially, symbolically, and "spiritually." Lived reality is complex; this aspect requires attention if we are to address structural barriers. Just as I was writing the conclusion, I witnessed a developing scenario. Ziba, with whom I had worked closely throughout my research, fell sick. Below is the script that she shared with me,

> I was seen by an oncologist. He told me that I had stage 4 cancer of the colon. I had six months to live. He said, "Do what you need to do. Take care of your Will and talk to your family about your wishes." I thought this was a heartless way to break the news that I was dying. He gave us the name of a counsellor that my husband, Ali, should visit. The oncologist told him, "You have to take care of yourself as this will be a tough time for you," You know, for over a year I have been telling my doctor of various symptoms, including severe back pain. He did not do any tests. He sent me to a physiotherapist. That was it.

After a couple of weeks, I learned that Ziba was administered such aggressive chemotherapy that she could barely walk or eat. How does one reconcile "news of impending death" with drastic attempts to reduce the onslaught of cancer? I am not passing judgment. I am wondering if Ziba received the news that she was going to die prematurely. Ali informed me that the family was going through a very difficult time. Ziba has two sisters who took care of her; her teenaged daughter blamed her father for not taking diligent care of her mother. Ali noted that they all have emotional moments when they cry a lot. Ziba has no other support. The rest of her family members are in Iran. The family has been given referrals, but they do not feel like phoning and do not know how to access the system they feel is overpowering.

The physician failed Ziba by dismissing her symptoms. The oncologist was only interested in breaking the news of terminal cancer without being sensitive to how the family would respond to their loved one dying at the age of fifty-two. The family's struggles building a new life in a country where they were racialized was of no interest to him. In other words, he did not consider their marginalized status and how this affected their ability to access a Eurocentric system of care (see, for example, Agnew 1998, 1997; Anderson 1996; and Spitzer 2011). How does one reconcile the contradiction of impending death with aggressive chemotherapy? Is the family being given hope that Ziba might live? If this is the case, why give news of death, and cause unimaginable grief and pain.

Ziba's case is not unique. Participants highlighted multiple ways in which they have been short-changed. Khadijah relayed that when her husband was admitted to a hospice facility, she was not informed that home hospice was a possibility. "I slept on the sofa in my husband's room for over a month. I developed back pain. It would have been easier if I was told that there is such a thing as homecare. When the doctor informed us about palliative care, he talked to my son. I was there but he did not even look at me." Did the physician think that a first-generation immigrant woman would not understand? Khadijah was an executive secretary with fifteen years of experience with an international organization in Nairobi (Kenya). Like her cohort, she was subject to de-skilling in the receiving country. Study participants understand palliative care to be a physical space of comfort and consolation at the end of one's life.

Death is a complex phenomenon linked with life.[3] A person's death requires reconfiguring social relationships, and for this to happen, socio-symbolic and spiritual dimensions are crucial; these dimensions are best realized in the context of social palliation, a caring society committed to the "cultivation of a humanitarian social imaginary" (Wilkinson and Kleinman 2016, 3). The foremost issue is that we are exploring an area that exists on an unequal plane, where most lives in today's world of neoliberal capitalism will remain "ungrieveable," to use Butler's (2004) term or may exist in "the zone of abandonment," to borrow Biehl's (2005) phrase. Though dismissed by the state and its institutions as "surplus bodies," Biehl's participants made "consistent efforts to communicate, to remember, to recollect and to write" (47), that the subjects of my study also recounted in the form of social wounding. I attribute their wounds to what I consider the existential condition of loneliness and isolation that have been normalized at the time when they are aging, having put in a lifetime's work in sustaining families across socio-political and geographical borders. Loneliness and isolation diminish one's humanity. This translates into a situation whereby one is not able to share one's life experiences of uncertainty and finitude – life and death. It is to this end that I advocate, as starting points, deep-level conversations for social palliation.

Paradigmatic Shift: Palliative Care to Social Palliation

A paradigmatic shift requires exploring large-scale societal forces and how these affect the everyday lived realities of socially marginalized people. In the case of our participants (first-generation immigrants), the societal force at work has been neoliberal capitalism. When Iranians and Ismaili-Muslims migrated to Canada in the 1970s and 1980s, this country was being embedded into the neoliberal system. Stanford (2014) puts it this way, "The last three decades have witnessed a far-reaching transformation of the Canadian economy, politics and culture. Canada is not unique in experiencing this neoliberal transformation, of course, but it has been as dramatic, thorough and socially destructive here as almost anywhere else in the industrialized world" (1). Neoliberalism is simultaneously a system of governance that fosters individualism and self-care, while absolving society from its responsibilities towards its citizens. Bone summarizes the outcome well (2012): "We have created a society in which materialism overwhelms moral commitment in which the rapid growth that we have achieved is not sustained environmentally or socially, in which we do not act together to address our common needs. Market fundamentalism has eroded any sense of community and has led to rampant exploitation of unwary and unprotected individuals" (657). In other words, "Neoliberal political and economic systems are also moral and ethical systems based on an ethic of individualization" (ibid.).

Commenting on gendered neoliberalism, Lindio-McGovern (2007) characterizes this global regime of governance as being the root cause of inequities and economic hardships, which affect immigrant populations the most. Especially pertinent is the regime's alliance with the nation-state. At the same time, she does not overlook immigrants' capacity to resist the system through self-definition and reconstruction of identities, along with challenging the parochial views of rights being confined within the unit of a nation-state.

Under the guise of "health reform," "retrenchment," and "community-based health," neoliberalism has eroded the health system, shifting the discourse from citizenship entitlement to self-care (Anderson et al. 1998; De Vos et al. 2015; Foley 2008; Ganti 2014; Misra et al. 2006; Pfeiffer 2008; Spitzer 2004). This shift has led to the burden of care falling on the families, particularly the women, who are considered "natural care givers." Han (2012) makes two points. First, neoliberal reforms put the onus for care onto families and individuals, "divesting the state of critical responsibilities for the well-being of its population" (3). Second, the discourses of self-care and self-responsibility that are advanced in health and social policy presume a self that is sovereign and morally autonomous" (ibid.). None of the palliative practitioners that I talked to discussed politics of care, that is, how downsizing and cost-cutting measures have compromised the principle of holistic and compassionate care. Volunteers, whose availability cannot be ensured, fill in gaps in social and emotional support. However, some suggestions have been put forward to combat the hegemony of biomedicine and its palliative care arm.

In her work on home care, for example, Bjornsdottir (2009) makes a case for nurses to reflect on the politics of downsizing and how this affects their care work. She urges the nurses to consider health services as an entitlement that would lead to a change of discourse from the market-model of outsourcing and privatization to affect-based care. Making a case for vulnerable populations who are subject to lifetime inequalities, Reimer-Kirkham et al. (2012) notes, "Most people share a common desire to approach the end of life in a peaceful and dignified manner, in the presence of loved ones, and filled with feelings of safety, comfort, and compassion. This echoes palliative care's goal which is to prevent and alleviate the pain and suffering of one of society's most vulnerable groups, the dying, and their family members" (1–2). The authors argue that no purpose is served if one's pain and suffering are recognized only at the end-of-life when one is about to die. Furthermore, they note, there is little research critically examining how social inequities and life circumstances shape how and where people die, and how they are cared for at the end of life. It is in this context that Wilkinson and Kleinman (2016) make a case for a caring society, whereby,

> Being cared for and caring for others is a necessary part of human life. We all have basic needs that can only be met through the kindness, help, and support of those who care for us. Particularly through the early and later years of life, the realization of human dignity is dependent upon the quality of care we receive. *Through care we are equipped to participate in social life, and in being cared for we are affirmed with recognition and value. In acts of care, real things are at stake, including life itself. In relationships of care we are made present to each other and are there for each other. Emotions are invested and worked through and become the grounds of interpersonal solidarity.* (161, emphasis added)

The above discussion captures the feelings and sentiments of study participants. As noted through the pages of this book, the latter felt abandoned and isolated as they aged and reached the end of their lives. They did not lay sole responsibility for their condition on their adult children. The participants are aware of the larger forces at work that I have articulated with reference to the neoliberal global capitalism that in many ways have molded their children for the labour force, leaving them little time to attend to their aging parents. The latter would agree with Wilkinson and Kleinman (ibid.) that one's life condition requires resolving societal issues. At the most basic level, social life should be "an enactment of substantive human values and thus it is inextricably moral and political" (162).

To reiterate the point made earlier, isolation and loneliness are existential issues. The majority of, but not all, participants experienced this condition on a varying scale. Others expressed anxiety as to what would happen as they grew old and their health failed them. They repeatedly informed me that their children were busy and would not be able to take care of them. Even if the children came forward and assured them that they would look after them, it was not agreeable to the aging parents. "We do not want to be a burden on them," is the aspect that they stated emphatically. At a deeper level, the issue was that the participants were rendered dependent by society. The discourse that they were exposed to was that they had to be taken care of as they aged; society did not "hear" the script that they could also be caring individuals and that they desired a caring society where social relations matter. And, as I have argued, it is in the context of social relationships that life and death can be addressed as one unit, a critical component of social palliation. It is important to emphasize that death is not always expressed in words; it constitutes the underlying script of a lived life.

The participants did not merely voice their concerns. Underpinning their stories is the determination to bring about change, which, in the context of this study, entails a shift from palliative care to social palliation. The contours of this shift constitute "slippages, openings, contradictions and possibilities for something different to emerge – but these have to be grounded in renovation and making critical an already existing activity" (Gramsci 1971, 330–1). A shift towards social palliation would translate into a caring society where one is not only cared for (dependency) but is positioned to offer intangible and affect-based care, that is reciprocal. This would require acknowledging one's life in the context of sociality. Social palliation is not exclusively confined to illness. It should be a generic part of social life.

In the above section, I have identified the workings of societal forces, foremost among them being neoliberal and racialized restructuring. These forces affect study participants' everyday lives, subjecting them, by and large, to isolation and loneliness. To reiterate, what the aging persons desire is sociality, which would allow them to affirm their personhood, allowing them to share their experiential knowledge on life and death, not in an abstract way but in relation to their lived realities. It is in this context that participants sought to create space for deep-level conversations through the prism of their sacred traditions. Examples of these are included, humbly, below because the heart-felt and affect-based nature of these traditions cannot be interpreted in absolute terms.

Sacred Traditions[4]

"Speak a new language so that the world will be a new one" (Rumi)[5]

As I worked on this manuscript, everyday I came upon an image: two stacks of books neatly placed on my bookshelf. The first stack was that of the ginanic tradition (lyrical meditative poetry) of the Shi'a-Ismaili Muslims in Gujarati. The second stack contained the English translation of classical Persian poets: volumes II and IV of Jalaludin Rumi's *Mathnawi'* (translated by Nicholson 1982); *Diwan* of Hafez (translated by Salehpour 1998), and the *Gulistan* of Sadi' (translated by Rehatsek 1998). These writers are famous for their mystical poetry, along with their scholarship on Islamic jurisprudence and theology, Arabic history, philosophy, and their exegesis of the Qur'an and the Hadith (sayings of the Holy Prophet Muhammed). Their works cross national boundaries and have influenced classical literature, especially in Turkey, Azerbaijan, Tajikistan, and Afghanistan.

Ginans: South Asian-Ismaili Melodies

The ginans are a body of religious poetry compiled in the twelfth and thirteenth centuries AD by several charismatic figures known as the *pirs*. The appeal of this tradition lies in its poetic, emotional, and melodious qualities. Constituting part of the living tradition, "they have long been a central part of the religious life of the [South Asian]/Nizari Ismaili community" (Esmail 2002; Virani 2011). The corpus is cherished because it contains "divine wisdom" on the meaning of life and death, highlighting qualities that could constitute part of social palliation. As Esmail (2002) has expressed it, "Perhaps the most potent source of poetic meditation is the experience of life and death" (63). Evoking how life and death are conjoined, he continues, "Life in certain forms comes to be seen as death and death metaphorically re-interpreted becomes a higher form of life" (63).

Classical Persian Poetry

Jalaludin Rumi, born in Tajikistan and raised in present-day Afghanistan, is well known for his soulful mystical poems, known at the *Mathnawi'*. Consisting of 27,000 lines (6 volumes), the *Mathnawi'* has been translated into English by R.A. Nicholson (1982). Some of Rumi's other major works include *Diwan-e Kabir* and *Diwan-e Shams-e Tabriz*. He also wrote in Turkish, Arabic, and Greek. Abu Muhammad Muslih al-Din bin Abdallah Shirazi, also known as Sadi' of Shirazi (1208–91) achieved fame as one of the greatest poets of the Persian literary tradition. He was well-versed in Islamic law, governance, history, Islamic theology, and Arabic literature. Two of his outstanding works are *Bustan* (The Orchard) composed in verse, and *Gulistan* (The Rose Garden), comprising prose (stories and anecdotes, for example, Mojaddedi 2009). Khwaja Shams-ud-Din Muhammad Hafez-e Shirazi (1315–90) is best known for his mystical poems composed in lyrics, an ideal mode for expressing the ecstasy of divine inspiration and love. Acclaimed throughout the Islamic world, his poems have inspired classical music, paintings, visual art, and calligraphy. His artistic legacy lives, evident in the visits paid by his devotees to his tomb in Shiraz and "Hafez Reading" circles in Iran and its diaspora.

The above texts were "neatly placed" on my shelf because I had not referred to them for a long time. Being an Ismaili-Muslim, I had been exposed to the Ginanic tradition from childhood and had the opportunity to listen to its lyrics in the Jamat Khana as well as at home, where selected verses were frequently recited as prompted on special occasions. Verses from the Persian literature were cited in English by some of my Iranian participants; others showed me Google-based translated verses. As living traditions, they are meant to be recited as opposed to merely being read. The texts of these sacred/mystical traditions on my shelf seemed to speak to me, stating that they contained a wealth of wisdom on the subject that I was writing on: living and dying and its interface with social palliation. I asked myself: "Would it not be wonderful if I were to use this resource to open space for deep-level conversations, a pathway for a more caring social world?" As I flipped through the pages of the texts, I realized that some of the verses that I read had been brought to light by study participants during our conversations. Their citations did not take place in a vacuum; they were grounded in real-life situations: the death of a loved one, the fragility of life, illness, crisis, and moments of mere reflections on life and death, along with social care in a new country. The appeal of these texts lies in their potential for generating conversations, notwithstanding differential, relational, and situational understandings of life and death expressed through the "the power of poetry and its linguistic beauty" (Esmail, 2002, 11). Referring to the binary of "religious" and "secular," Esmail (1998) notes, "From time to time, therefore, it is useful to free the mind of these kinds of categories and to *listen afresh to the language in which the basic dilemmas have been traditionally articulated*" (16, emphasis added). Furthermore, religious [sacred] thought and emotions, he argues, feed liberally on the human experience of the brevity and vulnerability of life on earth (64); see also Asani (2002). I recognized the value of "activating" the sacred texts, not in the form of exegesis but in relation to introducing the reader to "limits of language" to borrow a term used by the anthropologist Michael Jackson (2017). Jackson notes that it is only when we recognize such limits that we can acquire "new ways of understanding our-being-in-the-world, to new ways of connecting with others" (1). For him, these connections – a pathway for deep-level conversations – can lead to the realization that a single life is connected to other lives whereby the interplay between self and others assumes a trajectory of its own. Here, he argues, "The most intriguing thing about human relationships is that they include relations not only with other persons but with abstract ideas, imaginary beings and inert objects" (ibid.). These insights resonate with my take on sacred traditions.

In sum, my inclusion of the sacred traditions cherished by my interlocutors from the Canadian Ismaili-Muslim and Canadian-Iranian communities is informed by the search for alternative ways of being – that are not exclusively informed by neoliberal global capitalism, and are devoid of what Wilkinson and Kleinman (2016) refer to as "moral sentiment" and "with no sympathetic attachments to persons" (192). I would like to note that alternative ways of being do not constitute subjugated knowledge existing in its own orbit. I am interested in exploring how these traditions speak to restoring life conjoined with death, which are integral to social palliation.

I would like to emphasize that "the sacred" includes a lyrical appreciation of the world around us (for example, nature, the earth, and the universe and its galaxies). On a broader scale, the sacred addresses the question: What is it to live and what is it to die? This question was of critical importance for the study participants. Their experiences of living and dying have been subject to disruption in the wake of their loss of sociality; regenerating the latter amounts to death being understood as part of lived realities, because these unfold over a life course, as well as generationally. Given the richness of the verses from the Ginanic tradition and verses from the Persian poetry, it is my hope that I am modestly able to address one of the goals of anthropology: "to invoke neglected human capacities and to expand the limits of understanding and imagination" (Biehl 2015, 394). I share Bannerji's (1995) observation, "A whole new story has to be told, with fragments, with disruptions, and with self-conscious and critical reflections" (176). Equally relevant is Taussig's (1987) study on shamanism/healing in Colombia. Taussig makes three points. First, shamanism as a redemptive healing power benefits the colonizers as well, thereby creating space for social interactions between the Europeans and the Indigenous peoples. Second, presented as a montage of images and stories, shamanism invokes various possibilities and interpretations. Third, shamanism contains implicit social knowledge, and thus broadens our understanding of popular religion by emphasizing the ties between religion and medicine. Writing on the Yi minority in Southwest China, Mueggler (2001) also foregrounds the "shamanic chant" (poetic language) through which this community heals in the wake of state repression, prominent during the Great Leap Forward and the Cultural Revolution of the '60s. The sacred traditions introduced in this chapter perform a similar function, emphasizing that healing in the wake of social suffering and uncertainty of life does not take place in isolation or autonomously; it calls for an engagement with the larger society on the plane of social palliation.

I am mindful of the fact that the English rendition does not do justice to the wealth of wisdom included in the Indigenous languages, which include a combination of Gujarati, Sindhi, and Khojki dialects in the case of the Ginans, and Farsi, in the case of the Persian poetic corpus. Translated texts are the only way through which I can convey a modicum of the sacred texts cherished by the participants in varying degrees. At the same time, I write through the sounds, the rhythms, and poetic appeal of these languages, as Bannerji would express it (1995). My goal is to "open up" images and metaphors contained in the sacred texts to invoke the intricate connection between life and death with its potential for transformative change. I am aware that what I am sharing is a tiny and faint version of the corpus of the sacred texts, which calls for them to be recited as opposed to being inscribed on pages. Both traditions invoke a higher being (the divine), a term that lends itself to different interpretations based on how it resonates with the reader. It is my hope that these selected verses will serve to celebrate the heritage of minorities, which is not recognized otherwise, and in the process create space for foregrounding other sacred traditions. I am hopeful that the fragments from the sacred traditions will create space for us to listen and therefore act differently, allowing for more humane forms of living and dying. In these verses, death underpins life and is not severed from it. As Das and Han (2016) have expressed it, "life and death are folded together in the lives of individuals and communities" (1).

I have divided the following section into two parts. In the first part, I present verses in Gujarati and its oral interpretation by knowledgeable participants; in the second part, I include verses/stanzas from classical Persian poetry from two sources: the texts from my shelf as well as others suggested to me by participants, who referred to the Google to English translation. My reading of the verses includes "thematic orientations," which I hope will create space for reflection, a baseline for deep-level conversations on social palliation.

Glimpses of Ginanic Melodies

Part I

Tadhu(n) tadhu(n) mithadu(n) boliye
Gur gat ganga ne dware
Sarve sacheru thai ne chaliye
To saheb dil bhave

Two attributes emphasized in this verse are the need to speak in a sweet voice (*mithadu(n) boliye*) and to immerse oneself in truth (*sarve sacheru*). This is a pathway for endearment to the divine (*saheb dil bhave*).

~

Eji Sankdi sherimah mune Gur maliya
Mare loka su(n) vevar
Kanta ni mise Gurne namu(n)
Hathe karu(n) re parnam
I met the Divine (*Gur*) on a narrow street
But I must maintain my relationship with people
The only way I can pay homage to my Gur is by pretending that I am
    removing a thorn (from my foot).
This way I can bow and pay my respects

~

Eji dasi teri sami tere dar ubhi
Araj kare chhe hath, dasi chhu(n) teri

As your humble servant, I am standing in front of you
With my hands in supplication, I affirm that I am your humble servant

Eji hath jodine sami araj karu(n) chhu(n)
Hardam rahejo more sath, dasi chhu(n) teri

With my hands in supplication
Always remain close to my breath, I am your humble servant

Eji te din sami mune pas tedavjo
Pakdi lejo maro hath, dasi chhu teri

On that day (the day of my death) keep me close to you
Hold my hand, I am your humble servant

~

Ugamiya sohi din aathamiya
Hare fuliya sohi karmay
Chuniya mindar dhali pade
Hare janamiya sohi mar jai
Hare man bhamara tu lobhiyo

Hare maya mamate lobhano
Char divash kero pekhdo
Hare akhar khak ho jana

Just as the day has risen, it will set
The flowers that have bloomed will fade
The mansions that have been built will crumble
Those who are born will die
Why are you not generous and kind?
You are caught in the web of the material world
You are here for four days
Ultimately you will turn into ashes

Unchthi aayo bandeh neech kiyu dhiave
Chaar deen rahena bande jooth kiyu(n) kamave
Is re guneh bande kiya fal pave
Bharame mat bhoolo re bhai nami chaalo marna
Shafaayat rasool ki shaffayat paigamber ki
Jooth su(n) darna bhai jooth su(n) darna
Bhareme mat bhoolo re bhai nami chaalo marna

You descended from a high (*unch*) place to a low (*neech*) one
You will live for four days, why do you tell lies (*jooth*) [wrong-doing]
This kind of wrongdoing does not allow you to gather any fruits
In this material world, do not forget to act in a humble way
Rasool (the bearer of divine message) and the prophet are pure beings
Fear lies, fear lies [unrighteousness]
In this material world, do not forget to act in a humble way

Chāli chāli hu(n) thaki rahi
Swami hawe nahi(n) re chalay
Awagoon amara sami tame ma juvo
Sami have nahi(n) re rahevaay ....

Chedo nākhi ne sami dha(n)kajo
Awagoon ama tanaa aye
Ame to abadā aadhin chhu(n)
Lajā tamari ho rāya

I have walked and walked, I am now tired
My beloved one, I will not be able to walk anymore
Cover me with a "cloth" [give me shelter]
I am your "child"

Eji pak to sahebjinu(n) nam chhe
Tene jampiye sas usas
Dur ma dekho dil mahe vasay
Jem champa ful mahe(n) vās

Purity is the name of the divine
Meditate with your every breath
Do not look far
The divine resides in you like the scent in a flower

Eji sata ma chhodo mara munivaro
sata chhode pat jāya
Iman sarikho divdo
jene ajvade shah pāya

Dear brothers and sisters do not leave the path of truth
Those who abandon truth will go astray
Faith is like a lamp
In its light you will achieve the divine light

Eji raheni ajavadi Chanda su(n)
divasa ajavado surya
Tem ghat ajavado imansu(n)
Chau dise varase noor

The night is lit by the moon
The day is lit by the sun
In the same way your heart is lit by faith
Through this light, you will meet the divine (achieve your destination)

Eji marna hai re jaroor, jugmahe cheti ne chalo
Marna hai re jaroor

Death is a certainty. Tread carefully
Death is a certainty

(I am grateful to Jaff Valliani for editing
the transliteration of the Ginans)

Part II

The Reed: Jalaludin Rumi

Listen to the reed,
how it tells a tale
complaining of separation:
Ever since I was parted
from the reed-bed,
my lament has made
men and women weep.
I search for a heart
smitten by separation
that I may tell the pain
of love-desire.
Everyone who has got far from his source
harks back for the time
when he was one with it

(Jalaludin Rumi, *The Mathnawi*,
cf. Esmail 1998, 13)

"The first important thing in reading these lines is to forget what they state and try to listen to what they say. What I mean is the following. The poetry works on us: it strikes a chord, evokes something within us. Yet we cannot paraphrase it into a statement ... What the poetry evokes is a mystery, and without, on the other hand, simply assuming it as a 'mystery', it is more rewarding to inquire: what manner of speaking is this? What does it say about human language (and hence about human life)?" (Esmail, 14–15).

Calling upon the reader to reflect on Rumi's opening lines, Esmail continues,

The flute utters a sound, but it is more than a sound. It "tells" a tale, a story. The story speaks of an alienation, for the eloquence of the flute is heard only after its substance has been torn from its "source." In the reed-bed, all is silence. The separation precipitates lament; lament is a voice, where previously there was none. It is though language was born in anguish of a rupture. It is the sundering of being of which it speaks; and the paradox is that it is this sundering which is also the source of speech. (17)

Esmail observes that while "the anguish of severance is first voiced, we also hear undertones of a reassuring destiny – a healing of the breach. On one hand, there is a lost paradise. But thanks to the poetic imagination, there is also a faith, a hope which looking into the distance, sees paradise regained" (17).

Verses from Rumi

When you do things from your soul, you feel
   a river moving in you, a joy
Raise your words, not voice
It is rain that grows flowers, not thunder

Knock, And He'll open the door.
Vanish, And He'll make you shine like the sunFall,
And He'll raise you to the heavens.
Become nothing, And He'll turn you into everything.

Sadi' of Shirazi

A raindrop, dripping from a cloud
Ashamed when it saw the sea
"who am I, where is the sea? It said
As it saw itself from the eyes of humility
A shell embraced
it and made him a pearl

One who has vanity and conceit in his head
Imagine not that he will ever hear the truth

Human beings are members of a whole
In creation of one essence and one soul
If one member is afflicted with pain

Other members uneasy will remain
If you've no sympathy
For human pain
The name of humanity
You cannot retain

Deep in the sea
There are riches beyond your imagination
But if you seek safety
That is at the shore

Hafez

The mountain's face lifted me higher than
itself. A song's wink aligned me with joy. And a
tune paradise hums I came to know. The forest, letting me walk amongst its
    naked
limbs, had me on my knees again in silence
shouting – yes, yes my holy friend, let your
splendour devour me.

If your knees have not buckled in ecstasy while standing
when a veil parts. If a cherished tear of gratitude has not sung leaping from
your eye. If anything, your palm does touch cannot help reveal the
Beloved. My words are full of golden secrets that are not too hard
to crack and will remedy one hundred fears and ills.

Below is my reading of the verses (fragments) for further reflection.

Thematic Orientations

(a) The sacred traditions call for a way of listening that does not have
     a closure. In the process it does not conform to binaries such as
     them or us, rational or emotional, and affect or intellect.
(b) They recognize that life is fragile and uncertain.
(c) Glimpses of the corpus open space for an ethics of mutual care.
(d) They invoke the imaginative possibility of being awakened to
     human existence.
(e) They lead to the recognition of being-in-the-world, that is, social
     being as opposed to an exclusive biological self.

(f) They express existential issues of life along with the values by which it ought to be lived.

(g) Melodic words and rhythm embedded in these (and other) sacred traditions provide solace amidst the travails of life.

(h) They contain layered meanings that unfold in the context of lived and everyday realities.

(i) They bring home the intricate connection between life and death. "Life in certain forms comes to be seen as death and death metaphorically is re-interpreted, becomes a higher form of life" (reiterating for emphasis, Esmail 2002, 63).

(j) They address the paradox of the certainty of death and the uncertainty of life.

(k) Ultimately, they open the door for us to think in moral and ethical terms.

(l) By addressing the place of the sacred in human society, they continually revisit the question of the meaning of human life and death, articulated through a language of their own such as symbols and metaphors.

(m) They map pathways for alternative and more humane forms of life.

(n) Invariably, the sacred traditions have no limits to possibilities and imaginings. (I am reminded of Jackson's observation, "No matter how sophisticated our concepts become, they fail to do justice to the full range of human experience" (2016, 460).

(o) The significance of the sacred traditions may be recognized for their enabling capacity to address life situations during crises, including the contexts of everyday life.

(p) They constitute a powerful way of seeing "otherwise" (also refer to Taussig 1987).

Presenting fragments on the vernacular South Asian literature, the Canadian scholar Bannerji (1995) writes,

> Reader, you have just finished reading a piece put together by me from reading fragments of language, memories, textual allusions, cultural signs and symbols. It is clearly an attempt to retrieve, represent and document something ... You see, on the verge of writing, having written, I am still uncertain about the communicative aspect of it. (164)

I echo her anxiety about wanting to share it all but feel hesitant at the same time. Bannerji fears that what she has to say may end up "sounding stillborn, distant or abstract" (164). Yet, we need to communicate to overcome the binary framework of "us and them," that accords subjugated status to the traditions and literature of racialized minorities. To reverse this entrenched reality, we need to relay glimpses of the sacred traditions that Berardi (2017) refers to as the soul at work and "where the soul can be soulful again" (7) (also see Mueggler, 2001 and Taussig, 1987).

As I neared the end of this book, I asked myself, what last words could I convey to readers? I have sought foremost to establish hitherto unrecognized links between displacement and living and dying. Other than loss of livelihood and disruption of lives, the storied lives of study participants reveal a socially bare landscape relayed through their experiences of isolation and loneliness. For my participants, losing a social milieu reduced their capacity to share their understanding of life conjoined with death. For them, it was critical that they share this experiential knowledge with kith and kin and society at large. I came to this realization when participants did not feel the need to talk extensively about palliative care (institutionalized death severed from the life course, despite its focus on "dying with dignity"). In short, they did not take death as a discrete unit to be taken care of when someone passes away. As I have noted through the pages of *Social Palliation*, their barren social landscape is a function of their structural exclusion as racialized minorities, a situation exacerbated by neoliberal global capitalism. Ethnographic research invites us to investigate the inner recesses of everyday life affected by the larger forces at work. Participants' storied lives serve as illustrations. Stories elicit a response from readers and listeners. Participants came forward with the hope that their lived lives would ultimately make a difference, initiating what I refer to as deep-level conversations with readers and stakeholders. Here, sacred traditions as a means of starting such conversations can create a pathway for social palliation. Fundamentally, the latter enacts substantive human values, a caring society embedded in a world of social relationships.

As Stevenson (2014) observes, it is only when we make common cause with others that "we allow ourselves to be shaken, displaced from our customary dispositions and beliefs" (16). Capturing the spirit of the sacred fragments included above, she writes, "We are left to work out new ways to love, new ways to imagine the other that take this observation, that life is beside itself, seriously. Therein lies the ethical work of caring for ourselves and for others as imaginative beings, a task whose outlines cannot be traced in advance" (20).

The following anecdote (shared by Nizar Ramji, a friend) is of interest; it illustrates the paradigm shift towards social palliation, as enacted by a cab ride.

Cab Ride

I arrived at the address and honked the horn.
after waiting a few minutes.
I walked to the
door and knocked. "Just a minute," answered a
frail, elderly voice. I could hear something
being dragged across the floor.

After a long pause, the door opened.
A small woman in her 90's stood before me.
She was wearing a print dress
and a pillbox hat with a veil pinned
on it, like somebody out of a 1940's movie.

By her side was a small nylon
suitcase. The apartment looked as if no one had
lived in it for years. All the furniture was
covered with sheets.

There were no
clocks on the walls, no knickknacks or utensils
on the counters. In the corner was a cardboard
box filled with photos and glassware.

"Would you carry my bag
out to the car?" she said. I took the suitcase
to the cab, then returned to assist the woman.

She took my arm and we walked
slowly toward the curb.

She kept thanking me for my kindness. "It's nothing," I
told her. "I just try to treat my passengers
the way I would want my mother to be
treated."

"Oh, you're such a good
boy," she said. When we got in the cab, she gave

me an address and then asked, "Could you drive
through downtown?"

"It's not the
shortest way," I answered
quickly.

"Oh, I don't mind," she said.
"I'm in no hurry. I'm on my way to a hospice."

I looked in the rear-view mirror.
Her eyes were glistening. "I don't have
any family left," she continued in a soft
voice. "The doctor says I don't have very
long." I quietly reached over and shut off the meter.

"What route would you like me
to take?" I asked.

For the next two
hours, we drove through the city. She showed me
the building where she had once worked as an
elevator operator.

We drove through the neighborhood
where she and her husband had lived
when they were newlyweds. She had me pull up in
front of a furniture warehouse that had once
been a ballroom where she had gone dancing as a girl.

Sometimes she'd ask me to slow
in front of a particular building or corner and
would sit staring into the darkness, saying
nothing.

As the first hint of sun was
creasing the horizon, she suddenly said, "I'm
tired. Let's go now."

We drove in
silence to the address she had given me. It was
a low building, like a small convalescent home,

with a driveway that passed under a
portico.

Two orderlies came out to
the cab as soon as we pulled up. They were
solicitous and intent, watching her every move.
They must have been expecting her.

I opened the trunk and took the small suitcase to
the door. The woman was already seated in a
wheelchair.

"How much do I owe you?"
She asked, reaching into her
purse.

"Nothing," I said.
"You have to make a living," she
answered.

"There are other
passengers," I responded.

Almost without thinking, I bent and gave her a hug.
She held onto me tightly.

"You gave an
old woman a little moment of joy," she
said.
"Thank you."

I squeezed her
hand, and then walked into the dim morning
light. Behind me, a door shut. It was the sound
of the closing of a life.

I didn't
pick up any more passengers that shift. I drove
aimlessly lost in thought. For the rest of that
day, I could hardly talk. What if that woman had
gotten an angry driver, or one who was impatient
to end his shift?
What if I had refused to take the run,

or had honked
once, then driven away?

On a quick review,
I don't think that I have done anything
more important in my life.

We're conditioned to think
that our lives revolve
around great moments.

But great
moments often catch us unaware, beautifully
wrapped in what others may consider a small one.

To begin with, the above anecdote presents a moment that we can all relate to: calling a cab. We soon learn that the cab service is required by an older woman who is "noticed" by the driver to the extent of humanizing her (this rarely happens). He observes what she is wearing; at the same time, he notices that her life has come to a standstill. She has meagre belongings (small nylon suitcase) and her apartment looks as if no one has lived in it for years. She had covered her furniture with sheets, saying "goodbye," and through this gesture, goodbye to the world that had dismissed her humanity, that she was a person who had once a life and had contributed to society through her work as an elevator operator. Lack of acknowledgment of her life was poignantly revealed by the stark reality of a bare apartment (no cloaks, no utensils). Yet, in her own way she left traces of her personhood: photos and glassware placed in a cardboard box with the hope that someone might remember her. Critically important is the human relationship that develops between her and the cab driver. Taking her arm, he escorts her into the cab, establishing the kinship tie of "mother." The driver fulfills her wish to have one last look at the city that had taken no account of her aloneness and social suffering (ill and no one to take care of her). The driver's act of shutting off the meter and not charging her suggests his move out of the market-model and into the world of what I have referred to as social palliation. The hug and her holding on to the driver tightly suggest the kind of care that she must have aspired to living alone and isolated in her apartment. With the shutting of the door of the hospice, the driver recognizes that it was the sound of "the closing of a life." The scenario of an angry driver who could have driven away (not having the patience) points to the presence of an uncaring world. This example brings home the need for social palliation.

Appendix: Research and Methods

As I undertook this research, I was faced with three challenges. First, in keeping with the tenor of ethnographic research, I sought to identify a field site that would allow me to work with participants over an extended period. This concern drew me to further explore two communities with whom I have long-standing ties (Canadian-Iranians and Canadian Ismaili-Muslims). This focus made it possible for me to look at social palliation as a process rather than a defined field. I consider this to be critically important as this topic requires engaged conversations with stakeholders as well as study participants. I was mindful of the socio-cultural and systemic barriers that exist in the realization of a project whose orientation is "humanistic"; such a project requires critical awareness and nuanced analysis. In other words, I did not consider social palliation to be confined to one group or the other. Second, I wanted to delineate the parameters of palliative care that I found to be limiting owing to its connection with biomedicine; this was the case even though palliative care has expanded its reach to cover homes of patients as well as hospitals and nursing facilities. Third, I wanted to create space for study participants to share their storied lives in their own terms. This orientation includes non-discursive modes such as a repertoire of traditional knowledge (sacred traditions), participant observations, and the performance and enactment of everyday life events. More important, I wished to explore how participants re-make their worlds in the wake of suffering brought about by their status as racialized minorities; their suffering included factors such as deskilling of their credentials and structural exclusion, affecting intimate familial relations that resulted in participants' palpable experience of isolation and loneliness as they aged and neared death. Being severed from life, the issue of death loomed large.

I framed my research project and addressed the above issues as *social wounding*. I define social wounding as a mode of research that lends itself to a multilayered understanding of the lives of marginalized persons. Social wounding captures the workings of larger forces within the inner recesses of life. As such, it brings home the realities of what it is like to be displaced from a homeland and how life is reconfigured in the country of settlement. Furthermore, social wounding as a mode of ethnographic research speaks to multiple audiences: health professionals and other stakeholders, as well as readers interested in witnessing: What is it like to live and what is it like to die in a new land that does not acknowledge and affirm one's personhood? Rather than merely posing a question, social wounding contains seeds of possibilities and imagining another way of being that I have referred to as social palliation. As Gelya Frank (2000) has observed, "When readers engage with the life story [possibilities and imagining] and its various interpretations, *new meanings are created that will reverberate into readers' own local cultures and sometimes the dominant culture as well*" (23, emphasis added).

My task then was to identify participants willing to share their experiences of displacement, social wounding, and re-making of a world that addressed the core subject of this book: recapturing the conjoined unit of life and death and its implications for social palliation. Initially, British Columbia Hospice Palliative Care Association (BCHPCA) contacted me to conduct research on inclusive palliative care, a subject that participants did not wish to engage with on a large scale. Nevertheless, the BCHPCA helped me to establish initial contacts with palliative care practitioners; by means of the snowballing method, I had conversations with forty practitioners over the course of this research: from May 2015 to May 2018. Practitioners were happy to talk to me but, overall, they all foregrounded one script: the importance of palliative care for people with terminal illness. They emphasized compassionate and person- and family-centred care. I also attended three conferences and two workshops on palliative care. While presenters shared stories on how palliative care assists patients and their families, there was barely any critique of this system of care. More important, not much attention was given to the structural inclusion of racialized minorities.

My contact with research participants from the two communities (Canadian-Iranians and Canadian Ismaili-Muslims) was established through multiple channels noted in the introduction. Some participants talked to me at length, sharing their stories and life experiences, while others responded to my research topic briefly. Not wanting to restrict my project, I did not have a strict criterion except that I sought first-generation women and men, largely those who had migrated to Canada in the 1970s and 1980s. At the time of my research, participants were aging, having worked hard to raise families and make a life in Canada. Aging posed challenges as their career-oriented children had moved away or had adopted the host society's nuclear-family lifestyle. Feeling lonely and isolated, participants directed me to explore their stories of displacement and resettlement in a new country. The time span from early period of migration to the current period allowed me to explore the trajectories of their everyday lives. With the assistance of eight student- and community-based research assistants, I talked to fifty-five participants altogether, and engaged in dozens of hours of participant observations and informal conversations. Women came forward more than men; having been socialized into care work, the former felt that it was their responsibility to work towards more humane form of care (social palliation). The locations of my research (home, hospices, hospitals, nursing facilities, mosques, informal gatherings, cafeterias, and walking) were determined by the participants. As is the case with ethnographic research, I collected a substantive body of data: primarily field notes, transcribed and translated interviews (Farsi, Gujarati, and / or English), stories, anecdotes, and vignettes. Insights from this body of data informed my analysis on social wounding along with its embeddedness in re-making a world: storied lives (chapter 2), precarity as a resource for life (chapter 3), and re-making a home (chapters 4 and 5); here, the sacred traditions of the two communities proved to be crucial in expanding the horizons of participants' attempt to delineate a caring world (social palliation).

Participants discussed a range of issues such as life in the homeland, raising families in Canada, cooking, shopping, racism, aging, and the dilemmas and predicaments of everyday life, along with living and dying away from a homeland. Some women shared full stories; others profiled short summaries. Social palliation loomed large in a world where they experienced social injustice in terms of feeling "abandoned" as they aged and prepared for death. As I read and re-read the data, I noted the power of stories that participants shared with the understanding that one person's story reflects our collective border-crossing lives. I have fictionalized all names and changed identity markers in the interest of maintaining anonymity.

Methods must be viewed as part of epistemology: What is social knowledge for, how is it produced and for whom? Following my earlier work (2004), I have adopted a multifaceted approach. I have included mere description so that interested readers can visit field sites, imaginatively; I have engaged into analysis to provide a broader understanding of the forces at work and how these are re-configured by participants.

Last, I have sought to make space for the readers to interpret the data to foster dialogue and deep-level conversations. Here, sacred traditions lend themselves poignantly to achieving this goal as do stories relayed by the participants. Commenting on the role of stories, Gunaratnam (2013) observes that stories may be understood "as research methods, materials and as relationships" (159), stories restore "vitality to research and writing" (ibid.), and so do other alternative modes of articulation, which is the forte of ethnographic research.

Notes

Introduction

1 Jamila informed me that at times there were too many visitors, resulting in her grandmother not being able to rest or meditate.

2 Palliative care was the subject matter that British Columbia Hospice Palliative Care Association (BCHPCA) suggested I explore from the point of view of the inclusion of racialized minorities.

3 Displacement is not a one-time event. Its impact is felt continually in people's everyday lives. It is in this context that Das observes that an event can become "critical when it could not be subsumed within the existing repertoires of thought and action" (2007, 223). Narratives of displaced persons relay life circumstances and critical events not acknowledged by the host society. To address this omission, I suggest the framework of social palliation, a caring social milieu.

4 Anderson (1996) and Gunaratnam (2013), for example, have argued that "inclusive care" goes beyond culture; it must include socio-historical and political dimensions.

5 The relationship between displacement and social wounding can be gleaned from the loss of a milieu rich in human relationships where one is noticed as the bearer of familial history and country along with one's social identity. It cannot be overemphasized that it is within a network of relationships – lost through displacement – that one acquires a sense of belonging integral to which are conversations and lived realities of life and death.

6 Zimmermann (2012), for example, argues that palliative care discourse and practice promote acceptance of "a good death," whereby a patient is disciplined to die in a certain way. This orientation subjugates the lived realities of the dying.

7   BCHPCA did not participate actively in this research; they informed me that they had no funding.

8   Allison (2013) has noted "The quality of being needed is the first and most common use of the word human" (8).

9   It is important to note that participants were not nostalgic about the way of life they had left behind. What they missed was the complex world of social relationships not devoid of conflict.

10 Through its orientation to prolonged research and close encounters with the lives of the people, ethnography has played a key role in complicating the meaning of death in different societies. In her work in a shanty town in Brazil, Scheper-Hughes (1992), for example, documents the "letting go" of infants by mothers subjected to abject poverty as a form of "care." Such are the harsh realities of their lives brought about by corporate power. Stevenson (2014), in her work among the Inuit in Canada, presents a different scenario. She brings home the point that in this community, death is not an absolute certainty as the dead can continue to protect the living. This form of care emanates from connecting with the spirits, validating the presence of the souls and recognizing the existence of other species.

1 Research Context

1   Iran was not colonized by Western powers. This was because the country had regimes such as the Qazar dynasty (eighteenth century) and the Pahlavi dynasty (twentieth century, until 1979) that worked with Western powers, allowing them to extract the country's oil and gas resources.

2   Other South Asian communities also formed part of the exodus: the Sikhs, Parsees, Christians, and Hindus.

3   Unlike Iran, British colonization of Uganda was entrenched at multiple levels: militarized occupation, exploitation of resources and of labour, achieved at the cost of undermining the African way of life. After the country's independence in 1962, the colonial infrastructure of divide-and-rule remained intact, resulting in the Asian exodus.

4   This is a rough translation by way of introducing the reader to the images used in the ginans and the Iranian poetic tradition.

5   Despite regional and provincial differences, the ideology and practice of palliative care is common to all the provinces and territories within Canada's publicly funded health care system.

6   Abu-Lughod (2016) argues that the rights of Muslim women must be foregrounded in the wake of their countries' devastation by the imperialist West.

7   Although not all the references are pertinent to Islam, they are of theoretical import.

2 Storied Lives

1   I recognize that relations vary in terms of intensity. The critical issue is whether these relations include acknowledging lives that are not otherwise given recognition, as revealed in Saker's singular narrative, not unconnected to her cohort.
2   Ugandan Asians were given ninety days to leave the country. Upon their departure, their properties (homes and businesses) were confiscated.
3   It is interesting to note that through these activities Saker was seeking to shed her "refugee" status.
4   Canadian immigration policy admits four categories of people: family class, economic immigrants, refugees, and humanitarian cases.
5   Nazi, along with other women in my study, informed me that they were rarely hired to work in their area of qualification. They were primed to join the labour force through the buzz word of acquiring Canadian experience. This meant taking a position in the lower echelons of the workforce.
6   It is important to emphasize that the process of colonization has not come to an end. In the contemporary era, the colonizing global North continues to dominate the global South to the extent that the latter has not been able to free itself from its grip, which is exercised economically and militarily. As Kirmayer (2003) has observed, "Nor does the violence endured by the refugees [displaced persons] end with migration; it is embedded in the structures of most receiving societies" (181).

3 Precarity as a Resource for Life and Death

1   Life cannot be reduced to the level of bare survival. People seek to reaffirm their relational humanity (Biehl 2005; Berardi 2017; Garcia 2010; Stevenson 2004). This observation helps us to understand that death must not be reduced to mere physical extinction.
2   I wish to emphasize the point that while precarity is associated with suffering, it also nurtures the seeds for alternative ways of being (Allison 2013; Garcia 2010; Fischer 2010).
3   Conceptually there is a difference between precariousness and precarity. Precariousness refers to the social condition of exclusion, inequity, and

injustice. Precarity recognizes the agency of individuals exercised within socially marginalized spaces (Al-Mohammad 2016; Butler 2004, 2012; Shaw 2018).

4 Re-making a Home in the Diaspora

1 Home is understood as being connected to a wider world. It is this connection that leads to the affirmation of one's personhood, always in the context of sociality. As Al-Mohammad (2016) expresses it, "We are involved in the constant struggle to sustain and augment our being in relation to the being of others" (472); (also refer to Long, 2013).
2 Dossa (2019) cf. Riley and Paugh Ed. (190).
3 I have chosen to relay the experiences of differently abled persons, showing how the protagonists (includes Tamiza's story in chapter 5) effect a shift towards social palliation. The two stories (Firouzeh and Tamiza) are taken from my earlier work (Dossa 2009), condensed to include "narrative moments."
4 Low (2004, 2001, 2011) argues that we must not take space and place as a given. It is important that we engage with the question as to how the human quality of being needed is recognized and acknowledged, spatially and temporally. It is this aspect that Firouzeh highlights in her narrative – she must constantly negotiate a world that does not "see" her or "hear" what she has to say.
5 I wish to recognize Firouzeh's and Tamiza's work, both of whom undertake the task of nurturing their families; this context allows them to intervene in the reality that "in neoliberal regimes, the family has increasingly become the medical agent of the state" (Biehl 2005, 22). Their multiple negotiations of the service sector provide illustrative examples on what constitutes social palliation, in the wake of what Butler (1997) refers to as "enabling constraints." I concur with her insight that most systems have indeterminant elements; it is these elements that provide space for the subjects to negotiate (in this case) a Eurocentric system.

5 Negotiating Deep Divides: Foregrounding Social Palliation

1 Tamiza's attempt to imagine a community must be understood in relation to daily encounters not only with institutions but with the people who run these institutions.
2 Tamiza's efforts to access health and social services in the context of entitlements includes a larger goal, societal recognition of her children as human beings and not merely "disabled."

3 Tamiza's goal of social palliation may be understood in light of a situation where a neoliberal regime of care deprives one of social and citizenship rights. Cavarero (2000) puts it this way, "A unique individual is not the atomized individual of modern political doctrines. Instead the individual is unique not because she is free from any other; on the contrary, the relation with the other is necessary for her very self-designation as unique" (12, cf. Stevenson 2014, 246).

4 It is important to note that there were "success stories" whereby children took care of their parents. These were considered by participants as exceptional and not the norm. Recognizing the busyness of the lives of the children, parents were reluctant to be what one participant considered as being *mothaj* (dependent) on the children. Filial piety was no longer considered to be relevant in today's world of "meritocracy."

5 Names and all identity markers have been changed in the interest of anonymity.

Conclusion

1 In her work among the Inuit in northern Canada, Stevenson (2014) advocates a form of listening that allows us to pause and reflect on the words and life situations of the interlocutors. It is through this form of listening that she learned that death can be an ambiguous phenomenon. One can be dead but also alive, as indicated in the example of the raven who stayed around to guard the family in his role as an uncle.

2 Reader, through the pages of this book, you must have encountered multiple voices: study participants, practitioners, my summation of their narratives, as well as "voices" emerging from the sacred traditions. Through multi-voicing, I have sought to create space for your voice too. Hearing and listening to different voices (situational knowledge) is a viable pathway for social palliation.

3 I use the construct of social palliation to highlight the point that a caring society is not created in bits and pieces, such as institutional care or care offered during a crisis. I seek to draw attention to an organic form of caring where individuals and groups of people recognize the importance of mutual caring that includes but goes beyond caring in times of sickness or impending death. Here, one's life is conceived as embedded in a network of relationships. Bemoaning the loss of this social factor, Wilkinson and Kleinman (2016) observe, "Social inquiry was originally taken up as a vital matter with human interests at its heart; and by this standard it made no sense to argue that the study of society should be undertaken for the production of knowledge for its own sake and that its practitioners should operate from a position of moral detachment ... Over time, the

professionalization of social inquiry and its institutionalization within the academy took it away from these ameliorative and caring interests" (ix). It is to effect this shift that I suggest deep-level conversations as an ongoing venture. Kirmayer (2003) notes, "When the social worlds of patient and clinician are substantively different or unshared, the stories they tell each other may be mutually unintelligible" (168). In the same vein, Scheper-Hughes makes the critical point, "Human existence presupposes the presence of another" (1992, 23).

4 I am motivated to present sacred traditions because they open space for a fresh understanding of epistemological issues such as life and death and social palliation (organic caring). These fresh and new ways of understanding of our being-in-the world can facilitate deep-level conversations among groups of people who otherwise are separated; conversations that I advocate constitute edgework, to borrow the term from Brown (2005).

5 The elderly woman reminds us of Biehl's (2005) observation, "Our characters are those who might otherwise remain forgotten, and they want to be represented to be part of the matrix in which there is someone else to listen and to think with through their travails" (394).

References

Abdelhady, Dalia. 2008. "Representing the Homeland: Lebanese Diasporic Notions of Home and Return in a Global Context." *Cultural Dynamics* 20 (1): 53–72.

Abrego, Leisy. 2014. *Sacrificing Families: Navigating Laws, Labor, and Love across Borders*. Stanford: Stanford University Press.

Abu-Lughod. 2016. *Do Muslim Women Need Saving?* Cambridge: Harvard University Press.

– 1996. *Resisting Discrimination: Women from Asia, Africa and the Caribbean and the Women's Movement in Canada*. Toronto; Buffalo: University of Toronto Press.

– 1997. "The West in Indian Feminist Discourse and Practice." *Women's Studies International Forum* 20 (1): 3–19.

– 1998. "Tensions in Providing Services to South Asian Victims of Wife Abuse in Toronto." *Violence Against Women* 4 (2): 153–79.

– 2005. *Diaspora, Memory and Identity: A Search for Home*. Toronto, ON: University of Toronto Press.

Ahmed, Sara. 1999. "Home and Away: Narratives of Migration and Estrangement." *International Journal of Cultural Studies* 2 (3): 329–47.

Ahmed, Shahab. 2016. *What Is Islam: The Importance of Being Islamic*. Princeton: Princeton University Press.

Al-Mohammad, Hayder. 2016. "Never Quite Give: Calling into Question the Relation between Person and World in Post-invasion Iraq." In *Living and Dying in the Contemporary World: A Compendium*, edited by Veena Das and Clara Hans, 463–74. Oakland, California: University of California Press.

Allison, Anne. 2013. *Precarious Japan*. Durham: Duke University Press.

– 2016. Lonely Death: Possibilities for a Not-Yet Sociality. In *Living and Dying in the Contemporary World: A Compendium*, edited by Veena Das and Clara Hans, 662–74. Oakland, California: University of California Press.

Anderson, Joan M. 1996. "Empowering Patients: Issues and Strategies." *Social Science & Medicine* 43 (5): 697–705.

Anderson, Joan, and Sheryl Kirkham. 1998. "Constructing Nation: The Gendering and Racializing of the Canadian Health Care System." In *Painting the Maple: Essays on Race, Gender and the Construction of Canada*, edited by Veronica Strong-Boag, Sherill Grace, Avigali Eisenberg, and Joan Anderson, 242–61. Vancouver: University of British Columbia Press.

Arendt, Hannah. 1958. *The Human Condition*. Chicago, Illinois: University of Chicago Press.

Ariès, Philippe. 2013. *The Hour of our Death*. New York City: Vintage.

Asani, Ali. S. 2002. *Ecstasy and Enlightenment: The Ismaili Devotional Literature of South Asia*. London: I.B. Tauris Publishers.

Autism Society of America. 2000. http://www.autism-society.org.

Ayers, Alison J. and Alfredo Saad-Filho. 2015. "Democracy against Neoliberalism: Paradoxes, Limitations, Transcendence." *Critical Sociology* 41 (4–5): 597–618.

Bannerji, Himani. 1993. *Returning the Gaze: Racism, Feminism and Politics*. Toronto: Sister Vision Press.

– 1995. *Thinking Through: Essays on Feminism, Marxism and Anti-racism*. Toronto, ON: Women's Press.

– 2000. *The Dark Side of the Nation: Essays on Multiculturalism, Nationalism and Gender*. Toronto, ON: Canadian Scholars' Press.

Behar, Ruth. 1996. *The Vulnerable Observer: Anthropology That Breaks Your Heart*. Boston: Beacon Press.

– 2013. *Traveling Heavy: A Memoir In-between Journeys*. Durham, Duke University Press.

Benjamin, Walter. 1968. "The Storyteller: Reflections on the Work of Nicolai Leskov." In *Illuminations*. New York: Harcourt Brace & World, 83–109.

Berardi, Franco. 2017. *Futurability: The Age of Impotence and the Horizon of Possibility*. London; Brooklyn, New York: Verso.

Biehl, João. 2005. *Vita: Life in a Zone of Social Abandonment*. Berkeley: University of California Press.

Biehl, Richard. 2015. "Trauma in the Theater of the Body." In *Moving Consciously: Somatic Transformations through Dance, Yoga and Touch*, 109–23. Urbana, IL: University of Illinois Press.

Biehl, J. Guilherme, Byron Good, and Arthur Kleinman. 2007. *Subjectivity: Ethnographic Investigations*. Berkeley: University of California Press.

Billington, Tom. 2006. "Working with Autistic Children and Young People: Sense, Experience and the Challenges for Services, Policies and Practices." *Disability and Society* 21(1): 1–13.

Bjornsdottir, Kristin. 2009. "The Ethics and Politics of Home Care." *International Journal of Nursing Studies* 46 (5): 732–9.

Blevins, Dean, and Danai Papadatou. 2006. "The Effects of Culture in End-of-Life Situations." In *Psychosocial Issues Near the End of Life*, edited by J.L. Werth Jr and D. Blevins, 27–55. Washington, DC: American Psychological Association.

Boehm, A. Deborah. 2008. "'For My Children': Constructing Family and Navigating the State in the U.S.-Mexico Trans-nation." *Anthropological Quarterly* 81 (4): 777–802.

– 2012. *Intimate Migrations: Gender, Family, and Illegality among Transnational Mexicans*. New York: New York University Press.

Bone, John. 2012. "The Deregulation Ethic and the Conscience of Capitalism: How the Neoliberal 'Free Market' Model Undermines Rationality and Moral Conduct." *Globalizations* 9 (5): 651–66.

Bonny, Norton. 2000. *Identity and Language Learning: Gender, Ethnicity and Educational Practice*. New York: Longman.

Brah, Avtar. 1996. *Cartographies of Diaspora: Contesting Identities*. London; New York: Routledge.

Brown, Wendy. 2005. *Edgework: Critical Essays on Knowledge and Politics*. Princeton: Princeton University Press.

Butler, Judith. 1997. "Further Reflections on Conversations of Our Time." *Diacritics* 27 (1): 13–15.

– 2012. *Precarious Life: The Power of Mourning and Violence*. New York: Verso.

– 2012. "Precarious Life, Vulnerability, and the Ethics of Cohabitation." *The Journal of Speculative Philosophy* 26 (2): 134–51.

Byrne, Marjory. 2007. "Spirituality in Palliative Care: What Language Do We Need? Learning from Pastoral Care." *International Journal of Palliative Nursing*, 13 (3): 274–80.

Castillo, Rosalva Aida Hernández. 2012. "Cross-Border Mobility and Transnational Identities: New Border Crossings Amongst Mexican Mam People." *The Journal of Latin American and Caribbean Anthropology* 17 (1): 65–87.

Cavarero, Adriana. 2000. *Relating Narratives: Storytelling and Selfhood*. London: Routledge.

Cavell, Stanley. 1976. *Must We Mean What We Say*. Cambridge: Cambridge University Press.

Chatterjee, Ipsita. 2009. "Social Conflict and the Neoliberal City: A Case of Hindu-Muslim Violence in India." *Transactions of the Institute of British Geographers* 34 (2): 143–60.

Cheungsatiansup, Komatra. 2001. "Marginality, Suffering and Community: The Politics of Collective Experience and Empowerment in Thailand." In *Remaking a World: Violence, Social Suffering and Recovery*, edited by Veena Das, Arthur Kleinman, Margaret Lock, Mamphela Ramphele, and Pamela Reynolds, 31–73. Berkeley: University of California Press.

Coe, Cati. 2016. "Orchestrating Care in Time: Ghanaian Migrant Women, Family, and Reciprocity." *American Anthropologist* 118 (1): 37–48.

Colson, Elizabeth. 2003. "Forced Migration and the Anthropological Response." *Journal of Refugee Studies,* 16 (1): 1–18.

Constable, Nicole. 2014. *Born Out of Place.* Berkeley: University of California Press.

Crapanzano, Vincent. 2003. "Reflections on Hope as a Category of Social and Psychological Analysis." *Cultural Anthropology* 18 (1): 3–32.

Daftary, Farhad. 1990. *The Isma'ilis: Their History and Doctrines.* Cambridge England; New York: Cambridge University Press.

Daftary, Farhad, and Zulfikar Hirji. 2008. "The Ismailis: An Illustrated History." *Bulletin of the School of Oriental and African Studies* 72 (2): 401.

Daftary, Farhad, A. Sajoo, and S. Jiwa, eds. 2015. *Shi'a World: Pathways in Tradition and Modernity.* I.B. Taurus: London.

Das, Veena, 2003. *The Oxford India Companion to Sociology and Social Anthropology.* New Delhi; Oxford: Oxford University Press.

– 2007. *Life and Words: Violence and the Decent into the Ordinary.* Berkeley, Los Angeles, London: University of California Press.

– 2015a. "Naming Beyond Pointing: Singularity, Relatedness and the Foreshadowing of Death." *South Asia Multidisciplinary Academic Journal* 12: 1–16.

– 2015b. *Affliction: Health, Disease, Poverty* (Forms of Living). New York: Fordham University Press.

Das, Veena, and Renu Addlakha. 2001. "Disability and Domestic Citizenship: Voice, Gender, and the Making of the Subject." *Public Culture* 13 (3): 511–31.

Das, Veena, and Clara Han. 2016. *Living and Dying in the Contemporary World: A Compendium.* Oakland, California: University of California Press.

Datta, Ankur. 2016. "Dealing with Dislocation: Migration, Place and Home Among Displaced Kashmiri Pandits in Jammu and Kashmir." *Contributions to Indian Sociology* 50 (1): 52–79.

De Alwis, Malathi. 2004. "The Purity of Displacement and the Reterritorialization of Longing: Muslim Women Refugees in North-Western Sri Lanka." In *Site of Violence: Gender and Conflict Zones,* eds. Wenona Giles and Jennifer Hyndman, 213–31. California: University of California Press.

De Vos, Pol, and Patrick Van der Stuyft. 2015. "Sociopolitical Determinants of International Health Policy." *International Journal of Health Services* 45 (2): 363–77.

Dilworth-Anderson, Peggye, Gracie Boswell, and Monique D Cohen. 2007. "Spiritual and Religious Coping Values and Beliefs among African American Caregivers: A Qualitative Study." *Journal of Applied Gerontology* 26 (4): 355–69.

Dossa, Parin. 1985. "Ritual and Daily Life: Transmission and Interpretation of the Ismaili Tradition in Vancouver." Doctoral dissertation, University of British Columbia.

- 1999. "(Re)imagining Aging Lives: Ethnographic Narratives of Muslim Women in Diaspora." *Journal of Cross-Cultural Gerontology* 14 (3), 245–72.
- 2004. *Politics and the Poetics of Migration: Narratives of Iranian Women from the Diaspora*. Toronto: Canadian Scholars' Press.
- 2005. "'Witnessing' Social Suffering: Testimonial Narratives of Women from Afghanistan." *British Columbian Quarterly* 147: 27–49.
- 2009. *Racialized Bodies, Disabling Worlds: Storied Lives of Immigrant Muslim Women*. Toronto: University of Toronto Press.
- 2014. *Afghanistan Remembers: Gendered Narrations of Violence and Culinary Practices*. Toronto: University of Toronto Press.
- 2018. "From Displaced Care to Social Care: Narrative Interventions of Canadian Muslims." *American Anthropologist* 120 (3): 558–60.
- 2019. "Two Transnational Food Narratives." In *Food and Language: Discourses and Foodways across Cultures*, Kathleen C. Riley and Amy L. Paugh, 190–2. New York: Routledge.
- Dossa, Parin, and Cati Coe. 2017. *Transnational Aging and Reconfigurations of Kin Work*. New Brunswick, New Jersey: Rutgers University Press.
- Dunn, James R., and Isabel Dyck. 2000. "Social Determinants of Health in Canada's Immigrant Population: Results from the National Population Health Survey." *Social Science & Medicine* 51 (11): 1573–93.
- Duruz, Jean. 2005. "Eating at the Borders: Culinary Journeys." *Environment and Planning D: Society and Space* 23 (1): 51–69.
- Dyck, Isabel, and Parin Dossa. 2007. "Place, Health and Home: Gender and Migration in the Constitution of Healthy Space." *Health & Place* 13 (3): 691–701.
- Erel, Umut. 2009. *Migrant Women Transforming Citizenship: Life Stories from Britain and Germany*. Abingdon, Oxford, UK: Ashgate Publishing Group.
- 2011. "Reframing Migrant Mothers as Citizens." *Citizenship Studies* 15 (6–7): 695–709.
- Esmail, Aziz. 1998. *The Poetics of Religious Experience: The Islamic Context*. London; New York: I.B Tauris, in association with the Institute of Ismaili Studies.
- 2002. *A Scent of Sandalwood: Indo-Ismaili Religious Lyrics*. London, New York: I.B. Tauris.
- Fanon, Frantz 1963. *The Wretched of the Earth*. Grove Weidenfeld: New York.
- Farmer, Paul. 2003. *Pathologies of Power: Health, Human Rights, and the New War on the Poor*. Berkeley: University of California Press.
- Farr, Grant. 1999. *Modern Iran*. Boston: McGraw-Hill.
- Fassin, Didier. 2007. *When Bodies Remember: Experiences and Politics of AIDS in South Africa*. University of California Press.
- 2010. "Ethics of Survival: A Democratic Approach to the Politics of Life." *Humanity: An International Journal of Human Rights, Humanitarianism, and Development* 1 (1): 81–95.

– 2016. "The Value of Life and the Work of Lives." In *Living and Dying in the Contemporary World: A Compendium*, 770–83. Oakland, California: University of California Press.

Fischer, Michael MJ. 2010. "The Rhythmic Beat of the Revolution in Iran." *Cultural Anthropology* 25 (3): 497–543.

Fernando, Tisa. 1979. "East African Asians in Western Canada: The Ismaili Community." *New Community*: 361–8.

Foley, E. Ellen. 2008. "Neoliberal Reform and Health Dilemmas." *Medical Anthropology Quarterly* 22 (3): 257–73.

Frank, Arthur W. 1995. *The Wounded Storyteller: Body, Illness, and Ethics.* Chicago; London. University of Chicago Press.

Frank, Gelya. 2000. *Venus on Wheels: Two Decades of Dialogue on Disabilities.* California, University of California Press

Fry, Rosemary, Merryn Gott, Deborah Raphael, Stella Black, Linda Teleo-Hope, Hyeonjoo Lee, and Zonghua Wang. 2013. "Where Do I Go from Here? A Cultural Perspective on Challenges to the Use of Hospice Services." *Health and Social Care in the Community* 21 (5): 519–29.

Ganti, Tejaswini. 2014. "Neoliberalism." *Annual Review of Anthropology* 43: 89–104.

Garcia, Angela. 2010. *The Pastoral Clinic: Addiction and Dispossession along the Rio Grande.* Berkeley: University of California Press.

– 2016. "Medical, Legal, and Pharmaceutical Spaces: Death as a Resource for Life." In *Living and Dying in the Contemporary World: A Compendium*, 316–28. Oakland, California: University of California Press.

Gedalof, Irene. 2007. "Unhomely Homes: Women, Family and Belonging in UK Discourses of Migration and Asylum." *Journal of Ethnic and Migration Studies* 33 (1): 77–94.

Gilmartin, Mary, and Bettina Migge. 2015. "Migrant Mothers and the Geographies of Belonging." *Gender, Place & Culture* 23 (2): 1–15.

Good, Byron. 1994. *Medicine, Rationality, and Experience: An Anthropological Perspective.* Cambridge, UK; New York: Cambridge University Press.

Gramsci, Antonio. 1971. *Prison Notebooks.* Translated by Quintin Hoare and Geoffrey Nowell-Smith. Lawrence and Wishart: London.

Grande, Gunn, Kelli Stajduhar, Samar Aoun, Colleen Toye, Laura Funk, Julia Addington-Hall, Sarah Payne, and Todd Campbell. 2009. "Supporting Lay Careers in End of Life Care: Current Gaps and Future Priorities." *Palliative Medicine* 23 (4): 339–44.

Grewal, Inderpal, and Caren Kaplan. 1994. "Introduction: Transnational Feminist Practices and Questions of Post-Modernity." In *Scattered Hegemonies: Post-Modernity and Transnational Feminist Practices,* edited by Inderpal Grewal and Caren Kaplan, 1–33. Minneapolis and London: University of Minnesota Press.

Gunaratnam, Yasmin. 2013. *Death and the Migrant: Bodies, Borders and Care.* London and New York: Bloomsbury Academy.

Han, Clara. 2012. "Life in Debt: Times of Care and Violence in Neoliberal Chile." *POLAR: Political and Legal Anthropology Review* 36 (2): 358–9.
– 2016. "Echoes of a Death: Violence, Endurance, and the Experiences of Loss" *Living and Dying in the Contemporary World: A Compendium,* edited by Veena Das and Clara Han, 493–509. Oakland, California: University of California Press.

Hart, Gillian. 2008. "The Provocation of Neo Liberalism: Contesting the Nation and Liberation after Apartheid." *Editorial Board of Antipode* 40 (4): 678–705.

Higgins, Peter, and Fischer, Michael. 1981. "Iran: From Religious Dispute to Revolution." *American Anthropologist* 83 (2): 464–5.

Hill-Collins, Patricia. 2005. "Black Women and Motherhood." *In Motherhood and Space: Configurations of the Maternal through Politics, Home, and Body,* edited by Sarah Boykin Hardy and Caroline Alice Wiedmer, 149–59. New York: Palgrave Macmillan.

Hintzen, Percy C. 2004. "Imagining Home: Race and the West Indian Diaspora in the San Francisco Bay Area. *"Journal of Latin American Anthropology* 9 (2): 289–318.

Hua, Anna. 2005. "Diaspora and Cultural Memory." In *Diaspora, Memory, and Identity: A Search for Home,* edited by Vijay Agnew, 191–208. Toronto: University of Toronto Press.

Hussain, Yasmin, and Paul Bagguley. 2005. "Citizenship, Ethnicity and Identity: British Pakistanis after the 2001 'Riots'." *Sociology* 39 (3): 407–25.

Isin Engin. 2012. *Citizens without Frontiers.* New York: Continuum International Publication Group.

Isin, Engin, and Myer Siemiatycki. 2002. "Making Space for Mosques: Struggles for Urban Citizenship in Diasporic Toronto." In *Race, Space, and the Law: Unmapping a White Settler Society,* edited by Sherene H. Razack, 185–209. Toronto: Between the Lines.

Jack, Barbara A., J. Kirton, J. Birakurataki, and A. Merriman. 2011. "'A Bridge to the Hospice': The Impact of a Community Volunteer Programme in Uganda." *Palliative Medicine* 25 (7): 706–15.

Jackson, Michael. 2006. *The Politics of Storytelling: Violence, Transgression and Intersubjectivity.* Copenhagen: Museum Tusculanum Press, University of Copenhagen.
– 2011. *Life Within Limits: Well-being in a World of Want.* Durham: Duke University Press.
– 2016. *As Wide as the World Is Wise: New Directions in Philosophical Anthropology.* New York: Columbia University Press.

Joseph, Cynthia. 2013. "(Re)negotiating Cultural and Work Identities Pre- and Post-migration: Malaysian Migrant Women in Australia." *Women's Studies International Forum* 36: 27–36.

Kadar, Marlene. 2005. "Wounding Events and the Limits of Autobiography." *Diaspora, Memory, and Identity: A Search for Home,* 81–109.

Karim, Persis M., and Al Young. 2006. *Let Me Tell You Where I've Been: New Writing by Women of the Iranian Diaspora*. University of Arkansas Press.

Kittay, E. Feder. 2001. "When Caring Is Just and Justice is Caring: Justice and Mental Retardation." *Public Culture* 13 (3): 557–79.

Kirmayer, Laurence. 2003. "Failures of Imagination: The Refugee's Narrative in Psychiatry. *Anthropology & Medicine* 10 (2): 167–85.

Kleinman, Arthur, Veena Das, and Margaret Lock. 1997. *Social Suffering*. Berkeley: University of California Press.

Lamb, Sarah E. ed. 2009. *Aging and the Indian Diaspora: Cosmopolitan Families in India and Abroad*. Bloomington: Indiana University Press.

Lambek, Michael. 2016. "Afterlife." In *Living and Dying in the Contemporary World: A Compendium*, edited by Veena Das and Clara Han, 629–47. Oakland, California: University of California Press.

Lee, Jo-Anne. 1999. "Immigrant Women Workers in the Immigrant Settlement Sector." *Canadian Woman Studies* 19 (3): 97.

Li, Peter S. 2003. *Destination Canada: Immigration Debates and Issues*. Oxford: Oxford University Press.

Liebelt, Claudia, and Pnina Werbner. 2018. "Gendering 'Everyday Islam': An Introduction." *Contemporary Levant*, 3 (1): 2–9.

Lind, David, and Elizabeth Barham. 2004. "The Social Life of the Tortilla: Food, Cultural Politics, and Contested Commodification." *Agriculture and Human Values* 21 (1): 47–60.

Lindio-McGovern, Ligaya. 2007. "Conclusion: Women and Neoliberal Globalization Inequities and Resistance." *Journal of Developing Societies* 23 (1–2): 285–97.

Lock, Margaret M. 1993. *Encounters with Aging: Mythologies of Menopause in Japan and North America*. London: University of California Press.

Lock, Margaret M., and Judith Farquhar, eds. 2007. *Beyond the Body Proper: Reading the Anthropology of Material Life*. Duke University Press.

Long, Joanna C. 2013. "Diasporic Dwelling: The Poetics of Domestic Space." *Gender, Place & Culture* 20 (3): 329–45.

Low, Setha. 2004. *Behind the Gates: Life, Security, and the Pursuit of Happiness in Fortress America*. Routledge.

– 2001. "The Edge and the Center: Gated Communities and the Discourse of Urban Fear." *American Anthropologist* 103 (1): 45–58.

– 2011. "Claiming Space for an Engaged Anthropology: Spatial Inequality and Social Exclusion." *American Anthropologist* 113 (3): 389–407.

Low, Setha, and Sally Engle Merry. 2010. "Engaged Anthropology: Diversity and Dilemmas." An Introduction to Supplement 2 *Current Anthropology*, 51 (52): 5203–26.

Mahmood, Saba. 2012. *Politics and Piety: The Islamic Revival and the Feminist Subject*. Princeton: Princeton University Press.

Manderson, Lenore, and Pascale Allotey. 2003. "Storytelling, Marginality, and Community in Australia: How Immigrants Position their Difference in Health Care Settings." *Medical Anthropology* 22 (1): 1–21.

Malkki, Liisa H. 1995. *Purity and Exile: Violence, Memory, and National Cosmology among Hutu Refugees in Tanzania*. Chicago: University of Chicago Press.

– 2015. *The Need to Help: The Domestic Arts of International Humanitarianism*. Duke University Press.

Mankekar, Purnima. 2002. "'India Shopping': Indian Grocery Stores and Transnational Configurations of Belonging." *Ethnos* 67 (1): 75–97.

Mattingly, Cheryl. 2010. *The Paradox of Hope Journeys through a Clinical Borderland*. Berkeley: University of California Press.

McCarty, Teresa L. ed., 2011. *Ethnography and Language Policy*. New York, NY: Routledge.

McLean, Athena, and Annette Leibing. 2007. *The Shadow Side of fieldwork: Exploring the Blurred Borders between Ethnography and Life*. Malden, MA: Blackwell

Misra, Joya, Jonathan Woodring, and Sabine N. Merz. 2006. "The Globalization of Care Work: Neoliberal Economic Restructuring and Migration Policy." *Globalizations* 3 (3): 317–32.

Mobasher, Mohsen. 2016. *Iranians in Texas*. Austin: University of Texas Press.

Moghissi, Haideh, and Halleh Ghorashi, eds. 2010. *Muslim Diaspora in the West: Negotiating Gender, Home and Belonging*. Ashgate.

Modood, Tariq. 2005. *Multicultural politics: Racism, Ethnicity, and Muslims in Britain* (Vol. 22). Minneapolis: University of Minnesota Press.

Mojaddedi, Jawid. 2009. "The Gulistan of Sa'di: Bilingual English and Persian Edition with Vocabulary." *Bulletin of the School of Oriental and African Studies* 72 (3): 572–4.

Mueggler, Erik. 2001. *The Age of Wild Ghosts: Memory, Violence, and Place in Southwest China*. University of California Press.

Muehlebach, Andrea. 2012. *The Moral Neoliberal: Welfare and Citizenship in Italy*. University of Chicago Press.

Myerhoff, Barbara. 1980. *Number Our Days*. New York: Simon and Schuster.

Nicholson, Reynold Alleyne. 1982. *The Mathnawī of Jalālu'ddīn Rūmī*, Cambridge, England: E.J.W. Gibb Memorial.

Ong, Aihwa. 1995. "Making the Biopolitical Subject: Cambodian Immigrants, Refugee Medicine and Cultural Citizenship in California." *Social Science & Medicine* 40 (9): 1243–57.

Pandian, Anand, and M.P. Mariappan. 2014. *Ayya's Accounts: A Ledger of Hope in Modern India*. Bloomington, Indiana: Indiana University Press.

Pasura, Dominic. 2013. "Modes of Incorporation and Transnational Zimbabwean Migration to Britain." *Ethnic and Racial Studies* 36 (1): 199–218.

Pfeiffer, James, and Mark Nichter. 2008. "What Can Critical Medical Anthropology Contribute to Global Health?." *Medical Anthropology Quarterly* 22 (4): 410–15.

Phelps, Teresa Goodwin. 2004. *Shattered Voices: Language, Violence, and the Work of Truth Commissions.* Philadelphia: University of Pennsylvania Press.

Plaza, Dwaine. 2014. "Social Media as a Tool for Transnational Caregiving within the Caribbean Diaspora." *Social and Economic Studies* 63 (1): 25–56.

Povinelli, Elizabeth. 2011. *Economies of Abandonment: Social Belonging and Endurance in Late Liberalism.* Durham: Duke University Press.

Powell, Kathy. 2008. "Neoliberalism, the Special Period and Solidarity in Cuba." *Critique of Anthropology* 28 (2): 177–97.

Priestley, Mark. 1999. *Disability Politics and Community Care.* London: Macmillan.

Rahder, Barbara, and Heather McLean. 2013. "Other Ways of Knowing Your Place: Immigrant Women's Experience of Public Space in Toronto." *Canadian Journal of Urban Research* 22 (1): 145–66.

Ray, Oakley. 2004. "How the Mind Hurts and Heals the Body." *American Psychologist* 59 (1): 29.

Razack, Sherene. 1998. *Looking White People in the Eye: Gender, Race, and Culture in Courtrooms and Classrooms.* Toronto: University of Toronto Press.

– 2008. *Casting Out: The Eviction of Muslims from Western Law and Politics.* Toronto: University of Toronto Press.

– 2012. "Memorializing Colonial Power: The Death of Frank Paul." *Law & Social Inquiry* 37 (4): 908–32.

– 2014. "It Happened More Than Once: Freezing Deaths in Saskatchewan." *Canadian Journal of Women and the Law* 26 (1): 51–80.

Redclift, Victoria. 2016. "Displacement, Integration and Identity in the Postcolonial world." *Identites* 23 (2): 117–35.

Reimer-Kirkham, Sheryl Pesut, Barbara Sawatzky, Richard Cochrane, Marie Redmond. 2012. "Discourses of Spirituality and Leadership in Nursing: A Mixed Method Analysis.," *Journal of Nursing Management* 20 (8): 1029–38.

Reinders, Hans S. 2000. *The Future of the Disabled in Liberal Society: An Ethical Analysis.* Notre Dame: University of Notre Dame Press.

Riley, Kathleen, and Amy Paugh. 2019. *Food and Language: Discourses and Foodways across Cultures.* London and New York: Routledge.

Rehatsek, Edward. 1998. *The Gulistan or Rose Garden of Sadi'.* Tehran: Ibex Publisher.

Ross, Fiona. 2001. *Speech and Silence.* Berkeley: University of California Press.

Said, Edward. 1978. *Orientalism: Western Conceptions of the Orient.* London: Kegan Paul.

Salehpour, Saleh. 1998. *Diwan of Hafez.* Tehran: Booth Press.

Scheper-Hughes, Nancy. 1992. *Death without Weeping: The Violence of Everyday Life in Brazil.* Berkeley: University of California Press.

– 1994. "Embodied Knowledge: Thinking with the Body in Critical Medical Anthropology." *Assessing Cultural Anthropology* 229: 229–42.

Selby, Jennifer, Amelie Barras, and Lori G. Beaman. 2018. *Beyond Accommodation: Everyday Narratives of Muslim Canadians*. University of British Columbia Press: Vancouver.

Seymour, Jane, Sheila Payne, Alice Chapman, and Margaret Holloway. 2007. "Hospice or Home? Expectations of End-of-Life Care among White and Chinese Older People in the UK." *Sociology of Health & Illness* 29 (6): 872–90.

Shahidian, Hammed, and Asghar Fathi. 1992. "Iranian Refugees and Exiles since Khomeini." *Contemporary Sociology* 21 (3): 365–6.

Sharma, Sonya, and Sheryl Reimer-Kirkham. 2015. "Faith as Social Capital: Diasporic Women Negotiating Religion in Secularized Healthcare Services." *Women's Studies International Forum*, 49: 34–42.

Shaw, Jennifer. 2018. "'To Live My Life'": An Ethnography of Cross-border Life and Kinship from the Perspectives of Filipina/o-Canadian Youths." PhD dissertation, Simon Fraser University.

Smith, Joe, and Petr Jehlička. 2007. "Stories Around Food, Politics and Change in Poland and the Czech Republic." *Transactions of the institute of British Geographers* 32 (3): 395–410.

Somjee, Sultan. 2016. *Home between Crossings*. South Carolina: CreateSpace.

Spitzer, Denise L. 2004. "In Visible Bodies: Minority Women, Nurses, Time, and the New Economy of Care." *Medical Anthropology Quarterly* 18 (4): 490–508.

– 2011. *Engendering Migrant Health: Canadian Perspectives*. Toronto: University of Toronto Press.

– 2015. "Producing and Negotiating Non-Citizenship: Precarious Legal Status in Canada." *Contemporary Sociology* 44 (5): 662–4.

Stanford, Jim. 2014. "The Three Key Moments in Canada's Neoliberal Transformation." http://rabble.ca/columnists/2014/04/three-key -moments-canadas-neoliberal-transformation.

Stevenson, Lisa. 2014. *Life beside Itself: Imagining Care in the Canadian Arctic*. Oakland, CA: University of California Press.

Sugiman, Pamela. 2004. "Memories of Internment: Narrating Japanese Canadian Women's Life Stories." *Canadian Journal of Sociology/Cahiers canadiens de sociologie* 29: 359–88.

Taussig, Michael. T. 1987. *Shamanism, Colonialism, and the Wild Man: A Study in Terror and Healing*. Chicago, University of Chicago Press.

Thobani, Sunera. 2003. "War and the Politics of Truth-Making in Canada." *International Journal of Qualitative Studies in Education* 16 (3): 399–414.

– 2007. *Exalted Subjects: Studies in the Making of Race and Nation in Canada*. Toronto: University of Toronto Press.

– 2012. "Introduction and Thematic Orientations." *Race, Immigration and the Canadian State*. SA345-4-Study Guide, Simon Fraser University.

– 2014. "Performing Terror, Mediating Religion: Indian Cinema and the Politics of National Belonging." *International Journal of Communication* (19328036): 8.

– 2015. "Sovereignty, Culture, Rights: The Racial Politics of Gendered Violence in Canada." *Borderlands* 14 (1): 1–24.

Tsolidis, Georgina. 2011. "Memories of Home: Family in the Diaspora." *Journal of Comparative Family Studies* 42 (3): 411–20.

Vahabzadeh, Peyman. 2017. "Introduction: How to Approach This Book." In *Iran's Struggles for Social Justice*. Cham: Springer International Publishing, 1–7.

Virani, Shafique. 2011. *"Taqiyya* and Identity in a South Asian Community." *Journal of Asian Studies* 70 (1): 99–139.

Waltz, Mitzi. 2005. *Alternative and Activist Media*. Edinburgh University Press.

Warin, Megan, and Simone Dennis. 2008. "Telling Silences: Unspeakable Trauma and the Unremarkable Practices of Everyday Life." *The Sociological Review* 56 (2): 100–16.

Wendell, Susan. 1996. *The Rejected Body: Feminist Philosophical Reflections on Disability*. New York: Routledge.

Wiegratz, Jörg. 2010. "Fake Capitalism? The Dynamics of Neoliberal Moral Restructuring and Pseudo-Development: The Case of Uganda." *Review of African Political Economy* 37 (124): 123–37.

Wilkinson, Iain, and Arthur Kleinman. 2016. *A Passion for Society: How We Think about Human Suffering*. Oakland, CA: University of California Press.

Williams, Fiona. 2010. Migration and Care: Themes, Concepts and Challenges. *Social Policy and Society* 9 (3): 385–96.

Willis, Eliza, Christopher da CB Garman, and Stephan Haggard. 1999. "The Politics of Decentralization in Latin America." *Latin American Research Review* 34 (1): 7–56.

Yeates, Nicola. 2005. "A Global Political Economy of Care." *Social Policy and Society* 4 (2): 227–34.

– 2009. *Globalizing Care Economies and Migrant Workers: Explorations in Global Care Chains*. New York: Palgrave Macmillan.

Yee, May. 1993. "Finding the Way Home through Issues of Gender, Race and Class." In *Returning the Gaze: Essays on Racism, Feminism and Politics*, edited by Himani Bannerji, 3–37. Toronto: Sister Vision Press.

Zimmermann, Camilla. 2012. "Acceptance of Dying: A Discourse Analysis of Palliative Care Literature." *Social Science & Medicine* 75 (1): 217–24.

Zine, Jasmin. 2004. "Creating a Critical Faith-centered Space for Antiracist Feminism: Reflections of a Muslim Scholar-Activist." *Journal of Feminist Studies in Religion* 20 (2): 167–87.

– 2006. "Unveiled Sentiments: Gendered Islamophobia and Experiences of Veiling among Muslim Girls in a Canadian Islamic School." *Equity & Excellence in Education* 39 (3): 239–52.

– 2009. "Special Feature Article: Unsettling the Nation: Gender, Race and Muslim Cultural Politics in Canada." *Studies in Ethnicity and Nationalism* 9 (1): 146–63.

Index

www.ingramcontent.com/pod-product-compliance
Lightning Source LLC
Chambersburg PA
CBHW020252030426
42336CB00010B/726